THE UCSD HEALTHY DIET FOR DIABETES

THE UCSD HEALTHY DIET FOR DIABETES

A COMPREHENSIVE NUTRITIONAL GUIDE AND COOKBOOK

Susan Algert, M.S., R.D.

Barbara Grasse, R.D., C.D.E.

Annie Durning, M.S., R.D.

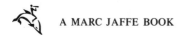 A MARC JAFFE BOOK

HOUGHTON MIFFLIN COMPANY   BOSTON   1990

For information about permission to reproduce selections from this book, write to Permissions, Houghton Mifflin Company, 2 Park Street, Boston, Massachusetts 02108.

Library of Congress Cataloging-in-Publication Data

Algert, Susan.
  The UCSD healthy diet for diabetes : a comprehensive nutritional guide and cookbook / Susan Algert, Barbara Grasse, Annie Durning.
     p.   cm.
  "A Marc Jaffe book."
  ISBN 0-395-49477-X
  1. Diabetes — Diet therapy — Recipes.   2. Diabetes — Nutritional aspects.   I. Grasse, Barbara.   II. Durning, Annie.   III. Title.
  RC662.A42   1990   89-20077
  641.5'6314 — dc20   CIP

Printed in the United States of America

S 10 9 8 7 6 5 4 3 2 1

Nutrient composition is based on The Nutrition Data System from The Nutrition Coordinating Center in Minneapolis, Minnesota, copyright © 1988.

"Herb and Spice Combinations," courtesy of the American Spice Trade Association. "Alternative Sweeteners," Phyllis A. Crapo, R.D. Originally published as "Available Alternative Sweeteners," Table 1, in "Use of Alternative Sweeteners in Diabetic Diet," *Diabetes Care,* vol. 11, no. 2, February 1988, p. 175. Reproduced with permission of the American Diabetes Association, Inc. Table 4, "The Cholesterol-Saturated Fat Index"; Figure 2, "Percent of Weight Lost on Various Reducing Programs"; and recipes for Crêpes, Falafel, Beer Batter Crust, and Zucchini Pie from *The New American Diet,* copyright © 1986 by Sonja L. Connor, M.S., M.D., and William E. Connor, M.D. Reprinted by permission of Simon & Schuster, Inc. Table 9, "How to Determine a Desirable Body Weight: 1983 Metropolitan Height and Weight Tables" and "How to Determine Your Frame Size," courtesy of Metropolitan Life Insurance Company. "Special 'Trim Line' Cuisine from Café Lautrec in La Jolla, California," courtesy of Café Lautrec. Table 13, "Frozen Desserts and Bars," reprinted from "Newsflash," September 1988, vol. 9, no. 5, a publication of the Diabetes Care and Education Practice Group of the American Dietetic Association. Table 16, "How to Make Food Adjustments for Exercise (Insulin-Dependent Diabetes)," © 1988 The American Diabetes Association, Inc., The American Dietetic Association. *Nutrition Guide for Professionals: Diabetes Education and Meal Planning.* Adapted from Marian J. Franz, *Diabetes and Exercise: Guidelines for Safe and Enjoyable Activity,* International Diabetes Center, © 1987, with permission from the publisher, Diabetes Center, Inc., Minnetonka, Minnesota. "Exercise Information for Persons with Insulin-Dependent Diabetes" and "Exercise Information for Persons with Non-Insulin-Dependent Diabetes," Marian J. Franz, M.S., R.D., C.D.E. Originally published as Tables 1 and 2 in *Diabetes Spectrum,* vol. 2, no. 4, September/October 1988, pp. 218–252. Reproduced with permission of the American Diabetes Association, Inc. Table 18, "The Quick Guide to Blood Glucose Levels," republished with permission from "Overcoming the Highs and Lows of Blood Glucose," by Janice L. Roth, R.N., B.S.N., C.D.E., *Diabetes Self-Management,* January/ February 1987. "Self-Monitoring Diary A." Developed by Hoechst-Roussel Pharmaceuticals, makers of DiaBeta®. "Self-Monitoring Diary B," Eli Lilly and Company, Indianapolis, Indiana 46038. Figure 3, "Time Action of Insulin," from *Managing Type II Diabetes,* by Arlene Monk, Sue Adolphson, Priscilla Hollander, Richard Bergenstal, International Diabetes Center, © 1988, with permission from the publisher, Diabetes Center, Inc., Minnetonka, Minnesota. Recipes for Banana "Ice Cream," Strawberry Dippers, and Pot Stickers, courtesy of Mary Donkersloot, R.D., nutrition counselor in private practice. Recipe for Salade Niçoise, courtesy of Café Champagne, John Culbertson Winery, Temecula, California.

To William and Sonja Connor for their many years
of hard work and dedication to the science of nutrition

ACKNOWLEDGMENTS

WE WOULD LIKE to thank the following individuals for their support and contributions. For recipe concepts and development, we extend thanks to Jo Bell, R.N.; Eva Brzezinski, B.S.; Mary Donkersloot, R.D.; Marylynne Rice, R.D.; and Nancy Stubblefield, M.S. Eva Brzezinski, B.S., and Cindy Toal, M.S., R.D., helped with manuscript preparation, nutritional analysis, and exchange calculations.

A number of people read the manuscript for technical accuracy. The material in Part One was reviewed by Jo Bell, R.N., Diabetes Research Coordinator, UCSD Medical Center; Christine Biby, R.N., B.S.N., F.N.P., C.D.E., Program Director, UCSD Diabetes Center; Orville Kolterman, M.D., Director, UCSD General Clinical Research Center, and Medical Director, UCSD Diabetes Center; Gayle Lorenzi, R.N., C.D.E., Coordinator, Diabetes Control and Complications Trial, UCSD School of Medicine; Mel Prince, M.D., Associate Director, UCSD Diabetes Center; Marylynne Rice, R.D., Pediatric Metabolic Nutritionist, UCSD Medical Center, and Nutrition Consultant, Whittier Institute, La Jolla; and Larry Verity, Ph.D., Director, Adult Fitness Program, San Diego State University. Lois Stanton, a free-lance food crafter in San Diego, reviewed the recipes. John Warwick contributed illustrations. And Evan Goldstein, coproprietor and master sommelier at Square One in San Francisco, contributed suggestions for wine accompaniments to our special occasion menus in Part Two.

Special thanks to David Rorvik, Proteus, Inc., for help with the writing of Part One, as well as to Phyllis Crapo, R.D., UCSD School of Medicine, Marion Franz, M.S., R.D., C.D.E., International Diabetes Center, and Sonja Connor, Research Associate Professor, Oregon Health Sciences University, for their inspiration and ideas. We would also like to acknowledge Donna Taylor and Van Jahnes Smith of the UCSD Business Office, Tom Antorietto of the UCSD Department of Medicine, and Cheryl Ward of the UCSD General Clinical Research Center for their valuable assistance in administrative matters.

CONTENTS

FOREWORD

ORVILLE KOLTERMAN, M.D.
MEDICAL DIRECTOR, UCSD DIABETES CENTER

As WE APPROACH the twenty-first century, dietary therapy has reached center stage in almost all segments of our society. This is true both for patients with specific disorders, such as diabetes, as well as for individuals who are interested in preserving their health.

At the same time that prudent dietary practices are being extolled, we are presented with many trendy culinary celebrations that fall far short of carefully considered guidelines recommended for healthful nutrition. Those of us who are committed to following sound dietary practices face a conflict. All too often, we end up feeling that we must make a choice between healthful practices and "socially desirable" behavior.

At times, the peer pressure can be tremendous. Patients frequently come to view their dietary prescription as a strict list of exclusions, which, if implemented, make them stand out. They feel punished and begin to resent the dietary regimen.

In essence, this dilemma represents a failure on the part of health care providers. We are able to tell patients what they should and should not do, but we have not been able to provide them with the necessary tools to follow prescribed dietary guidelines. *The UCSD Healthy Diet for Diabetes* addresses this deficiency.

This book is, in effect, a dietary workshop for those with diabetes mellitus. First, the authors discuss the basis for current dietary recommendations so that patients and their families can understand the rationale behind them. In addition, the book provides helpful pointers collected from clinical experience regarding ways of incorporating needed changes into the routines of daily living. Finally, and most important, the cookbook concludes with a finale of prudent, varied, and delicious recipes that embrace our dietary recommendations, yielding dishes that are, at once, healthful, tasty, and attractive.

In fact, most of the recipes introduced here will find general acceptance — so that other family members and friends will want to partake of the same menu. What a pleasant turnaround for the diabetic diet — to be sought after, rather than feared. Enjoy!

PART ONE

THE NEW NUTRITION:
GREAT TASTE
AND GOOD HEALTH

1

THE HEALTHFUL GOURMET ALTERNATIVE: MODIFICATION, *NOT* DEPRIVATION

WHY *THIS* COOKBOOK IS THE BEST CHOICE FOR YOU

Overheard

FIRST WOMAN: "Did you know Ellen was just diagnosed as having diabetes?"

SECOND WOMAN: "Oh, no! How awful. I really feel for her. You know how she loves to cook."

FIRST WOMAN: "And *eat!* And think of her boys and her husband. I grew up in a home with a diabetic father, and, believe me, they're going to have to get used to *bland* and *boring* real quick."

SECOND WOMAN: "There go all those wonderful desserts."

FIRST WOMAN: "No more wine. You know how Ellen loves a little wine. And you can say goodbye to all those great sauces."

SECOND WOMAN: "You can say goodbye to *all* of Ellen's great dinners — *period.*"

No you won't. *Not* if Ellen chooses *this* cookbook. Our recipes, based on the most up-to-date and medically sound research, make the diabetic days of bland and boring a thing of the past. We offer exciting new culinary fare that will please *every* member of the family and promote good health in both diabetics and nondiabetics alike.

We believe this is an important new cookbook for *all* people with diabetes and their families to own. We offer the most varied and least restrictive recipes possible — without sacrificing any health benefits. We are able to do this because we are fortunate to be in a research setting that provides leading-edge knowledge about diabetes and nutrition. Many of the foremost experts in these fields are on our team.

3

Lack of knowledge and creativity has resulted in too many cookbooks that don't meet the needs of people with diabetes. Our cookbook is a valuable addition to the market of diabetes cookbooks. Few offer as many resources as we do — a wealth of dietary advice, weight loss tips, menu ideas, fast-food information, and over 200 recipes to challenge and excite the palate. These recipes represent a new, lighter, more healthful style of eating for *everyone* to enjoy.

SPICE IS THE VARIETY OF LIFE (AND GOOD FOOD)

We're fortunate to be in one of the great culinary meccas of the world. Southern California has become a kind of melting pot of international and nouvelle cuisines, where great food is not merely created and consumed but is also celebrated.

Every recipe in this book has been tested not only clinically and scientifically in the research kitchen, but also in the kitchens and on the tables of countless individuals. Whether the menus you select from this book feature foods that are Californian, Mexican, Chinese, French, German, Indian, Italian, Middle Eastern, Far Eastern, South American, or vegetarian, you can be certain they not only have passed rigorous standards for nutritional value but also have passed many pleased — and discriminating — palates.

Part of the secret of our success is that we never deprive. We don't expect you to make radical changes in your eating style. Instead, we *modify* not only standard all-American favorites but also the great cuisines of the world to make them compatible with the nutritional needs of the person with diabetes. We have become highly adept in the art and science of *substitution*. We rarely take away without giving back at the same time.

And what we give back — in place of excesses of fats, sugars, salts — provides satisfaction without worry of risk. We have, through long trial and error, learned how to use herbs and spices that effectively compensate for "missing" salts and other flavors characteristic of so many unhealthful foods. We have learned how to substitute "missing" sugars with other healthful alternatives. We have become, as one of our patients put it, "culinary con artists" when it comes to serving up richly textured, full-flavored recipes and meals largely devoid of excessive fat.

This book takes you on a culinary trip around the world — offering such dishes as moussaka, cassoulet, gazpacho, and seafood creole. The diverse cultures represented here emphasize meat as a condiment, focusing on starches, such as beans, rice, or pasta, as main courses. They use a far wider variety of seasonings than do traditional American cooks. Each country or region has its own special flavors — cumin and cilantro from Mexico; basil, oregano, and garlic from Italy; and curry from India, just to name a few.

As for those who were worried that they would no longer be able to experience great meals at Ellen's table, we offer the following reassurances. If Ellen chooses this cookbook, her friends can look forward to such items as Banana Smoothies, Garlic Lover's Dip, Black Forest Mushrooms, French Onion Soup, Spicy Seafood Wontons, Hearty Lamb and Barley Stew, Watermelon Salad with Raspberry Vinegar, Blueberry Cobbler, Ginger-Lemon Broccoli, Red Cabbage with Apples, Frijoles Refritos, Spanish Rice, Delhi Delite, Snapper Creole, San Diego Cioppino, Party Sushi Rolls, Melon with Slivered Almonds and Ginger, Baked Halibut with Cilantro-Citrus Sauce, Chicken Artichoke Pie, Chicken Marsala with Mushrooms, Shrimp and Feta à la Grecque, Cauliflower Curry, Beef and Bean Chili, Veal Parmesan, Pumpkin Rolls, Garlic Cheese Casserole Bread, French Toast Bake, Beef Teriyaki, Spinach Dill Phyllo Triangles, Chocolate Mousse Pie, Santa Fe Blue Cornmeal Bread, Strawberry Dippers, and Cream Puffs. And these regional and international menus will give Ellen some great ideas for luncheons and dinners.

All-American
New England Soup
Picnic Potato Salad
BBQ Chicken
Applesauce Cupcakes

French
French Onion Soup
Spinach Salad with Sprout Dressing
Zucchini Boats
Chicken Breasts Dijon
Chocolate Mousse Pie

Italian
Basil and Tomato Salad
Italian Vegetables
Chicken Marsala with Mushrooms
Fruit Medley

Middle Eastern

Toasted Pita Chips
Tabbouli
Falafel, with Tahini or Yogurt Dressing

Mexican

Fiesta Bean Salad
Spanish Rice
Frijoles de la Olla
Fish Tacos
Burritos de Manzana

Indian

Lentil Soup
Cauliflower Curry
Delhi Delite
Harvest Fruit with Yogurt Dressing

Southwest Buffet

Spicy Salsa with No-Fry Tortilla Chips
Easy Bulgur Pilaf
Baked Halibut with Cilantro-Citrus Sauce
Santa Fe Blue Cornmeal Bread
Strawberry Dippers

German

Red Cabbage with Apples
German Potato Bake
Beef Roulade
Low-Calorie Chocolate Pudding

Neither Ellen nor her family and friends may have to give up even the wine. Many diabetics (see our discussion of meals and wines for special occasions, pages 51–57) can drink wine in moderation, based on the recommendations of the American Diabetes Association. We have asked an internationally known wine steward to provide suitable selections for some of our menus. Don't worry. We've asked him to pick wines that properly complement our cuisine and please the palate without bankrupting the pocketbook.

Meanwhile, there's still more good news for Ellen (and all readers of this cookbook). Even many of the most exotic of our gourmet meals fall into our Quick or Easy categories. At least a third of our recipes can be prepared and/or assembled in less than 30 minutes, many in less than 20.

WEIGHT CONTROL, DISEASE PREVENTION, AND LONG-TERM MAINTENANCE

There are additional benefits to be derived from this book. Obesity is a problem many of us have to contend with. It is, in itself, a disease, and it contributes significantly to a number of other diseases. People with body weights that are 20 to 40 percent, or greater, above their optimal weight are much more likely than those with optimal weight to develop diabetes. So, for people with diabetes, weight control is especially important.

The typical diabetes cookbook largely ignores this crucial issue. We have devoted enormous amounts of time and resources to developing the richest taste and texture in our recipes for the fewest number of calories. Each of our recipes will contribute to an overall eating style that will help you shed excess pounds and *keep them off.*

We offer you a special chapter on weight control. We discuss different types of weight loss diets, the importance of body fat distribution, and what to do to correct your weight problem. After all is said and done, there is really only *one* scientifically and medically sound way to lose weight and keep it off permanently, and we tell you what that is.

We also provide you with a number of useful tips on dining out and entertaining friends. As we've already indicated, we've made it easy for you to invite guests for dinner without having to apologize for bland and boring meals. In another special chapter, we tell you how you can dine out at restaurants healthfully. We even provide you with guidelines on selecting foods at McDonald's, Wendy's, and other fast-food franchises.

Good nutrition has two partners that also play a role in overall diabetes management — exercise and medication. In fact, the diabetes treatment triad represents a balance between the three components of diet, exercise, and medication. In the final two chapters we have provided a brief discussion of the relative importance of these two other components of diabetes management. We highlight the benefits and risks associated with exercise and provide you with an overview of blood glucose monitoring and management.

2

THE BASICS: THE GOALS AND HOW TO ACHIEVE THEM

GENERAL NUTRITIONAL GOALS FOR PEOPLE WITH DIABETES

Diabetes mellitus is the third most serious disease in the United States, and its incidence is estimated to have increased tenfold in the past forty-five years. Diabetes is characterized by an abnormally high blood glucose (sugar) level that is caused by a disruption in the process by which the body's cells convert glucose to energy. The incidence and prevalence of diabetes and its complications becomes more widespread daily. Close to 6 million Americans are diagnosed as having diabetes. Another 5 million or more still do not know they have it.

The disease diabetes mellitus has two major forms, each with its own characteristics and symptoms, as defined in Table 1. Type I (*insulin-dependent*) diabetics make up about 10 percent of all cases. By far the most severe of the two types, it can occur at any age, but usually appears in childhood. This individual is unable to produce enough of the hormone insulin to metabolize food properly and needs to follow both a dietary and medication regimen for successful treatment.

The overwhelming majority (approximately 90 percent) of the diabetic population have *non-insulin-dependent,* or Type II, diabetes. It often appears after the age of forty. It is characterized by resistance to insulin and poor utilization of the hormone rather than by lack of the hormone. This form of diabetes is very strongly associated with obesity, sedentary lifestyle, and advancing age.

No matter what type of diabetes you have, there are three gen-

Table 1 Diabetes: The Two Major Types

	Insulin-Dependent Diabetes	Non-Insulin-Dependent Diabetes	
	Type I	Type II — Nonobese	Type II — Obese
Disorders	Secrete no insulin	Secrete some insulin but not enough to control blood glucose	Secrete some insulin; body is unable to use insulin properly.
Treatments	Daily insulin injections, exercise, and healthful diet; oral hypo-glycemic agents do not work.	Insulin is a key treatment for many (along with exercise and a healthful diet); oral hypoglycemic agents sometimes work.	Weight loss and exercise; insulin and oral hypoglycemic agents sometimes work.
Onset	Sudden	Variable, slow or sudden	Usually slow
	Usually occurs in childhood or adolescence.	Usually develops after age 40, but may occur earlier.	Usually develops after age 40.
	Common symptoms are extreme thirst and hunger, frequent urination, and rapid weight loss.	Symptoms vary; mild cases may have no symptoms; severe cases may have many symptoms seen in Type I.	Infection that won't go away is often the first sign; may also experience extreme thirst, hunger, and need to urinate.

eral goals related to nutrition, based on the recommendations of the American Diabetes Association.

1. Maintain appropriate levels of glucose and fats in the blood. It is the balance in the body among the amount of insulin, the amount and type of food you eat, and your exercise that determines blood glucose and blood fat (cholesterol and triglyceride) levels. The goal is to keep blood glucose as stable as possible to prevent the metabolic imbalance that results from blood sugars that are too high (hyperglycemia), or insulin reactions, a condition that results from blood sugars being too low (hypoglycemia). Specifically, the goal is to match the amount of food you eat with the amount of insulin in your body, whether your body still produces insulin on its own or whether you need insulin injections or pills. Stable control of blood glucose levels will enhance your feelings of well-being.

Diabetes is often associated with high levels of cholesterol and triglyceride in the blood, substances that increase the risk of heart disease. People with diabetes are at a greater than average risk of developing heart disease. Changing your diet to decrease fat and cholesterol intake, thus lowering your blood fat levels, can substantially reduce this risk.

2. Maintain consistency in meal planning (nutrient intake and timing of meals) if you have insulin-dependent diabetes. Stress weight management if you have non-insulin-dependent diabetes.

If you have Type I, or insulin-dependent, diabetes, consistency in meal planning is of vital importance. Eat your meals at approximately the same time every day. And the amount and types of food you eat at each meal should be about the same from day to day. Your insulin dose is based on the food that you eat and on your activity level. A meal plan based on the exchange lists developed by the American Diabetes Association (see chapter 5) will help you plan your diet while giving you variety and consistency. Consistency in food intake will help your food and insulin work together to regulate your blood glucose at optimal levels.

A large majority (60 to 90 percent) of the people with the far more common, Type II, non-insulin-dependent, diabetes are overweight. For these people the most important dietary principle is weight control to help the body make the best use of its own insulin. We'll discuss the specifics of weight management in a subsequent chapter.

3. Alter your diet to limit salt, fat, sugars, and alcohol while increasing the intake of complex carbohydrates (starch and fiber).

This goal includes consuming a diet lower in total fat, saturated fat, and cholesterol, and higher in the polyunsaturated and monounsaturated fats than the usual American diet. Lowering the percentage of total calories derived from fat will, of necessity, increase the percentage of calories derived from other sources. The American Diabetes Association recommends replacing fat calories with carbohydrate calories. It is important, though, that these be the right kind of carbohydrates, the "complex" type. It is equally important to control your intake of carbohydrates in the form of refined or processed sugars, such as table sugar or sucrose. We'll have more to say, shortly, about carbohydrates, fats, and protein, but for now we simply want you to know that the best diet for a person with diabetes is a low-fat diet that has a normal protein content, a reduced content of refined or processed sugars, and an increased content of complex carbohydrates (starches). In addition, the diet should include relatively large amounts of dietary fiber. We'll have more to say about fiber in this chapter as well. Table 2 compares the composition of the typical American diet with the dietary recommendations of the American Diabetes Association.

ACHIEVING THE GOALS

The basics of good nutrition apply to everyone, including those with diabetes. A knowledge of nutrition basics is a key element in the successful management of the disease.

All food is made up of nutrients, substances that supply the body with the biological fuel it needs to grow, to maintain and repair itself, and to regulate its many complex functions and processes. The fifty or so nutrients needed by the body to stay healthy are divided into two general groups: macronutrients and micronutrients.

The macronutrients are nutritional factors that the body needs in relatively large amounts: the proteins, fats, and carbohydrates. Let's look at those first and see what we need to do to get the appropriate amounts of each into our daily diet.

PROTEIN

We need protein to build, maintain, and repair body tissues and to assist in a number of body functions. A protein molecule is a long chain of smaller units called amino acids. The arrangement of the amino acids in the chain distinguishes one protein in a food from an-

Table 2 Typical American Diet vs. Recommendations of the American Diabetes Association

Food Group/Nutrient	Typical American Diet	American Diabetes Association Recommendations
Carbohydrate	45% of total calories	Up to 60% of total calories
Complex and naturally occurring sugars	25% of total calories	All or nearly all of the total carbohydrate
Refined and processed sugars	20% of total calories	Modest intake within the meal setting; consult physician or dietitian for amount
Protein	15% of total calories	.8 g/kg body weight
Fat	40% of total calories	30% of total calories
Saturated	15% of total calories	10% of total calories
Monounsaturated	16% of total calories	10% of total calories
Polyunsaturated	6% of total calories	10% of total calories
Cholesterol	400–500 mg per day	300 mg or less per day
Dietary Fiber	15–20 g per day	Up to 40 g per day
Sodium	4–6 g per day	2–3 g per day

other. The protein in egg white, for example, is qualitatively different from the protein in wheat. When you eat protein, it is broken down into amino acids during digestion and then recombined by cells to form the specific proteins that the body needs.

The body needs all twenty-two of the amino acids to function properly. There are eight amino acids (nine for infants) that the body cannot make itself and that we must get from food. These eight are called the *essential* amino acids. Foods that have all eight of these in the proportions needed by the body are said to contain a *complete protein*. These foods have more nutritive value than a food with incomplete protein which is either missing one of the essential amino acids altogether or has an inadequate amount. Complete proteins generally come from animal sources, such as meat, fish, eggs, cheese,

Table 3 Complementary Protein

Combinations	Recipes
1. Rice and legumes	Red Beans and Rice*
2. Rice, wheat, and soy	Tofu Spread* on whole wheat bread with rice cakes
3. Rice and sesame seed	California Wild Rice* with fruit and nuts (use sesame seeds instead of pecans)
4. Rice and milk	Delhi Delite Easy Rice and Cheese Casserole*
5. Wheat products and milk	Cheesy Broccoli and Pasta* Angel Hair Sauté* Calzones* Pasta Pie Italiano*
6. Wheat and beans	Falafel and Falafel Dressings (with pita bread)
7. Cornmeal and beans	Santa Fe Blue Cornmeal Bread* and Frijoles de la Olla*
8. Beans and milk	Chilaquiles topped with Frijoles Refritos* and skim-milk cheese
9. Peanuts and milk	Apple Snacks* with nonfat milk

*Recipes in Part Two

and milk. Most proteins from plant sources are incomplete but can be combined appropriately to make a complete protein containing a balanced amount of the essential amino acids. Table 3 shows how incomplete proteins from the plant kingdom complement one another in nutritious combinations.

For most Americans, complementing proteins is not a problem. In fact, most of us consume *too much* protein, particularly animal protein. Our daily consumption often tops 20 percent of our total calories, whereas our actual needs are much lower. We recommend getting between 12 and 20 percent of your daily calories in the form of protein. Eating more protein than you need means that the excess calories will be used for energy or stored as fat.

If you follow our other recommendations, your protein requirements will take care of themselves. You will consume less animal protein and more plant protein, and the effect will be positive, not only on your health, but also on your wallet!

Table 4 The Cholesterol–Saturated Fat Index (CSI)

	CSI	Calories
Fish, Poultry, Red Meat (3½ oz or 100 g cooked)		
White fish (cod, halibut, snapper, sole, perch)	4	91
Shellfish (clams, oysters, scallops)	4	91
Tuna (canned, packed in water)	4	91
Salmon	5	149
Shellfish (shrimp, crab, lobster)	6	104
Poultry, no skin	6	171
Beef, pork, and lamb:		
10% fat (ground sirloin, flank steak)	9	214
15% fat (ground round)	10	258
20% fat (ground chuck, pot roast)	13	286
30% fat (ground beef and pork, lamb steaks, ribs, pork and lamb chops, roasts)	18	381
Cheese (100 g or 3½ oz)		
Low-fat cottage cheese, pot cheese	1	98
Part-skim mozzarella	12	256
Cheddar, Swiss, Monterey Jack, American	26	386
Eggs		
Whites (3)	0	51
Egg substitute (equivalent to 2 eggs)	*	91
Whole (2)	29	163

FAT

Dietary fat, once it enters the body, helps form cell membranes, and supplies essential fatty acids and fat-soluble vitamins that are needed for various functions (but that the body cannot manufacture). Fat also cushions and supports internal organs, such as the heart, lungs, and the skeleton.

Americans have adopted a high-fat diet in a big way, primarily because fat enhances the flavor and texture of many foods. Our actual requirement is for only about 1 tablespoon of fat per day, yet many Americans consume a 40 to 50 percent fat diet that translates into 6 to 8 tablespoons of fat per day. Unfortunately, a great deal of this fat comes from animal sources and saturated vegetable fats that are unhealthful. Additionally, high-fat foods are very dense in calories. Fat is the most concentrated source of calories. By weight, fat contains

	CSI	Calories
Fats (¼ c or 4 T)		
Peanut butter	5	353
Most vegetable oil	8	530
Mayonnaise	10	431
Soft vegetable margarine	10	432
Hard stick margarine	15	432
Soft shortening	16	530
Very hydrogenated shortening	27	530
Butter	37	430
Coconut oil, palm oil, cocoa butter (chocolate)	47	530
Frozen Desserts (1 c)		
Ice, sorbet	0	245
Sherbert or low-fat frozen yogurt	2	290
Ice milk	6	214
Ice cream, 10% fat	13	272
Rich ice cream, 16% fat	18	349
Specialty ice cream, 22% fat	34	684
Milk Products (1 c)		
Skim milk (0.1% fat) or nonfat yogurt	*	88
2% milk or plain, low-fat yogurt	4	144
Whole milk (3.5% fat) or whole-milk yogurt	7	159
Sour cream	37	468
Imitation sour cream	43	499

*Less than one

more than twice as many calories as protein or carbohydrate. One gram of fat contains more than 9 calories, whereas 1 gram of carbohydrate or protein contains only 4 calories.

Health experts agree that Americans can substantially lower their risk of heart disease by eating less total fat, particularly by eating less saturated fat and cholesterol. Saturated fat is found primarily in animal products and in three fats from the plant kingdom — coconut, palm, and cocoa (or chocolate). Cholesterol is another type of dietary fat that is found only in animal products, such as meat, poultry, fish, eggs, and dairy products. Cholesterol in foods works along with saturated fat to elevate a person's blood cholesterol level, and an excess of both cholesterol and saturated fat can clog the arteries, including the ones serving the heart.

Researchers at the University of Oregon have devised a Choles-

Table 5 Oils and Fats

Choose oils (and margarines made from oils) that are higher in polyunsaturated and/or monounsaturated fat. Strictly limit or avoid those that are high in saturated fat.

| Type of Oil or Fat | Percent of Total Fat | | |
	Polyunsaturated	Monounsaturated	Saturated
Safflower oil	74	12	9
Sunflower oil	64	20	10
Corn oil	58	24	13
Vegetable oil (soybean and cottonseed)	48	30	18
Canola (rapeseed)	32	62	6
Peanut oil	30	46	19
Chicken fat	21	45	29
Vegetable shortening	15	51	32
Lard	12	45	40
Olive oil	9	74	14
Beef fat	4	42	48
Butter	4	23	61
Palm oil	2	11	81
Coconut oil	2	6	86

Source: United States Department of Agriculture Human Nutrition Information Service

terol–Saturated Fat Index (CSI) to make it easier for people to select foods that are low in *both* saturated fat and cholesterol. In Table 4, the lower the CSI number, the better the food choice for the prevention of heart disease. Foods with lower CSIs are also better choices for those who are overweight, because they are generally lower in calories.

We recommend, along with the American Diabetes Association, that you decrease your total fat intake to 30 percent or less per day. Fats in foods are a mixture of saturated and unsaturated fats. Saturated fats should comprise no more than 10 percent of total fat calories. The other 20 percent should come from the two types of unsaturated fat — poly- and monounsaturated fat. Table 5 lists the different fats and oils in our foods and the types of fat they contain.

We have known for a long time that polyunsaturated fats lower blood cholesterol levels. However, monounsaturated fat has recently received a great deal of publicity because population studies from the Mediterranean region show a lower incidence of heart disease in spite of higher blood cholesterol levels and a high intake of fat. The type of fat consumed in this area is primarily olive oil, one of the monounsaturated fats. Clinical studies in the United States have shown that the vegetable oils high in monounsaturated fat may be as beneficial as the polyunsaturated fats in lowering cholesterol levels when consumed in large quantities.

But consuming large quantities of monounsaturated fats is not the best way to lower your cholesterol because they are also concentrated sources of calories and can cause you to gain weight. The best advice is to maintain a lower fat diet (30 percent of total calories or less), making sure that the types of fat you eat are either monounsaturated or polyunsaturated vegetable oils. So, deciding to use safflower or walnut oil (both primarily polyunsaturated) or olive or peanut oil (both primarily monounsaturated) in a recipe is really a matter of personal preference. You will find that olive oil is a popular ingredient in many of our recipes because of the unique flavor that it lends to many foods.

The fats found in fish oils and seafood are highly polyunsaturated and contain a group of substances called the omega-3 fatty acids. Research has shown that these fats may be useful in lowering blood levels of cholesterol and triglycerides in *nondiabetic* individuals. However, preliminary studies show that the fish oils may actually *worsen* low-density lipoprotein (LDL) cholesterol (see the Glossary of Dietary Terms) levels and glucose control *in persons with diabetes.* As a result of the initial research, some people have begun buying fish oil capsules and indulging in large amounts of shellfish (crab, shrimp, and lobster). Neither of these practices is advisable. The safety and efficacy of the fish oil capsules, particularly cod liver oil, which contains excessive amounts of vitamins A and D, has not been established. What you should do is follow the recommendations for a low-fat, low-cholesterol diet. Eat fish (not shellfish) *at least three times per week* in quantities of *3 to 4 ounces per serving.* Shellfish is recommended one to two times per week, but not more often, in 3- to 4-ounce portions. Shellfish contains more cholesterol than ordinary fish.

Table 6 shows you how to modify the typical American diet to make food choices that are lower in fat and cholesterol.

Table 6 Cutting the Fat and Calories from Your Diet

Typical American Diet	Teaspoon Fat	Lower-Fat Alternatives	Teaspoon Fat
Breakfast:			
Poached egg with	1	Quick Pita Breakfast*	½
2 strips bacon	1		
2 slices toast with	0		
2 t margarine	1½		
1 T jam	0		
1 c orange juice	0	1 small orange	0
Snack:			
1 c coffee	0	1 c coffee	0
1 doughnut	2	Apple Oatmeal Muffin* with 1 t margarine and 1 T dietetic jelly	1½
Lunch:			
Deli sandwich:			
2 slices rye bread	0	California Chicken Sandwich*	1½
2 oz turkey	1		
2 oz cheese	3½		
1 T mayonnaise	2		
Tomatoes, lettuce			
½ c coleslaw	1½	Picnic Potato Salad* (½ c)	½
1 oz potato chips	2		
1 apple	0	1 small apple	0
1 c whole milk	1½	1 c low-fat milk	1

Typical American Diet	Teaspoon Fat	Lower-Fat Alternatives	Teaspoon Fat
Snack:			
1 oz Doritos	2	No-Fry Tortilla Chips* (12–16) with ⅓ c Guacamole*	2½
Diet soda	0	Diet soda	0
Dinner:			
8 oz broiled steak	4	3 oz Poached Salmon with 4 T Spinach Sauce*	1½
Baked potato with 1 t butter and 1 T sour cream	0 1½	Easy Bulgur Pilaf* (½ c)	1
Tossed salad with 1 T Thousand Island dressing	0 1½	Italian Vegetables* (½ c) with 1 t margarine	1
1 c chocolate ice cream	6½	Melon with Slivered Almonds and Ginger*	½
Iced tea with sugar	0	Sugar-free iced tea	0
Snack:			
2 chocolate chip cookies	1	Cereal Crunch* (1 c)	1
1 c whole milk	1½	Spiced Cocoa* (¾ c)	0
Total Teaspoons Fat:	33½ (or 11 tablespoons)	**Total Teaspoons Fat:**	12½ (or 4 tablespoons)
		Total Teaspoons Fat Saved:	21 (or 7 tablespoons)
Total Calories: 3400 % Calories Fat: 44		Total Calories: 2000 % Calories Fat: 29	

*Recipes in Part Two

The following recommendations were developed by the U.S. Department of Agriculture to help people avoid too much fat, saturated fat, and cholesterol in their diets:

1. Choose lean meat, fish, poultry, dried beans, and peas as protein sources.
2. Use skim milk or low-fat milk and milk products.
3. Moderate your use of egg yolks and organ meats (reserve for special occasion or once a week at most).
4. Limit your intake of fats and oil, especially those high in saturated fat, such as butter, cream, lard, heavily hydrogenated fats (some margarines), shortenings, and foods containing palm and coconut oils.
5. Trim fat off meats.
6. Broil, bake, or boil rather than fry.
7. Moderate your use of foods that contain fat, such as breaded and deep-fried foods.
8. Read labels carefully to determine both amount and type of fat present in foods.

Fat Substitutes   New "fat substitutes" will soon be hitting the food market. They have been developed to meet the ever-increasing demand for a product that functions as a fat in foods and yet contains fewer calories than the fats we have been discussing. Simpless is one of these fat substitutes that was put on the market in early 1988. It is made from protein and hardens when heated so that it cannot be used in baking and frying foods. However, it is found in many desserts, such as ice cream and chilled pies, and in salad dressings. The Food and Drug Administration (FDA) is currently reviewing another new fat substitute made from sucrose polyesters, called Olestra, for its safety and efficacy. Olestra is not degraded by heat and contains no calories because the body does not absorb it. It will probably be added to foods such as shortenings and oils. Consumers will see many new fat substitutes in the next few years, depending on FDA investigation and approval. Your dietitian is the best person to help you fit them into your food plan.

CARBOHYDRATES

Carbohydrates are the main source of energy for the body. They come in three general forms — *simple, complex,* and *fibers.* Simple carbohydrates, including sucrose (table sugar), fructose (fruit sugar), lactose (milk sugar), and sweeteners such as corn and maple syrup, are made up of one or two sugar molecules. Complex carbohydrates are larger molecules that occur mainly as starches. Potatoes, pastas, breads, rice, and vegetables are all complex carbohydrates. Fibers are similar to starches and complex carbohydrates but are not digestible in the human body. (They do, however, serve several useful purposes in the body.)

Americans are similar to people in the rest of the world in that they derive most of their calories from carbohydrates. They differ, however, in that they get a good deal of their carbohydrates from refined or processed sugars. The average American gets one fifth to one fourth of daily calories in the form of refined sugars. Historically, people with diabetes have been told to avoid consuming refined sugars, which were thought to cause extreme ups and downs in blood glucose levels. However, recent research suggests that lower intakes of refined sugars may not be as harmful for people with diabetes as was once believed. This is not to say that refined sugar is not going to have an effect on your blood glucose level. All foods will affect blood glucose whether they contain protein, fat, or carbohydrate. The bottom line is that you must maintain good blood glucose control when you eat foods containing refined sugars. Intake of table sugar and foods containing table sugar and other sweeteners need to be controlled and substituted for other foods in the diet in a reasonable way to maintain a desirable weight. If you choose an occasional treat, try to eat something that is nutritious as well as sweet. Check the list of foods for occasional use that accompany the exchange lists in chapter 5. We recommend that you do not exceed one serving per day of these foods.

Hidden sugars are hard to avoid in our food supply. Some catsups and salad dressings actually contain about 30 percent sugar! Some of the prepared mixes for coating and baking meat and chicken are more than 50 percent sugar! Sugar is also added to some peanut butters, hot dogs, luncheon meats, breads, pickles and relishes, mayonnaise, crackers, etc. The only way to avoid consuming hidden sugar is to become an avid label reader.

When checking food labels, beware of "natural" sugars that are supposedly superior, or better for you, than sucrose or table sugar. Sucrose, which comes from sugarcane, is just as natural as the fructose and glucose found in honey, the fructose found in fruit, or the lactose found in milk.

Table 7 Types of Fiber

	Soluble	*Insoluble*
Type	Gums, pectins, mucilages, some hemicelluloses	Cellulose, lignin, some hemicelluloses
Sources	Legumes, oat bran, some fruits (prunes, figs, dates)	Whole grains (wheat, barley, corn, rye), vegetables, some fruits (lemons, raspberries, blackberries)
Function	Lowers blood cholesterol; stabilizes blood sugars; increases efficient use of insulin by the body	Absorbs water, which helps prevent constipation; enhances intestinal function

Fiber Content of Selected Foods (Soluble and Insoluble)

Food	Serving Size	Grams Fiber	Major Type of Fiber
Kidney beans	½ c	5.8	Soluble
Pinto beans	½ c	5.7	Soluble
Lentils	½ c	2.7	Soluble
Black-eyed peas	½ c	4.9	Soluble
Oat bran	⅓ c	4.2	Soluble
100% Bran cereal	⅓ c	9.1	Soluble
Oatmeal	¾ c	2.7	Soluble

The ideal type of carbohydrate for the person with diabetes is starch or *complex* carbohydrate. Americans currently consume 25 percent of their calories as complex carbohydrates and naturally occurring sugars (i.e., fruit). As recommended by the American Diabetes Association, your goal should be to increase your intake of these complex carbohydrates to 50 to 60 percent of your total calories.

Foods that are high in complex carbohydrates generally contain a great deal of fiber as well. Fiber, which has traditionally been known as "roughage" or "bulk," is the portion of foods that is not digested in the small intestine. Fiber is found in fruits, whole grains, and vegetables. Researchers at the University of Kentucky School of Medicine have shown that when fiber is consumed as part of a high-

Fiber Content of Selected Foods (Soluble and Insoluble)

Food	Serving Size	Grams Fiber	Major Type of Fiber
Prunes	⅓ c	5.8	Soluble
Fiber One cereal	⅓ c	11.9	Insoluble
Grapenuts	¼ c	2.2	Insoluble
Shredded Wheat	⅔ c	3.4	Insoluble
Wheaties	1 c	2.6	Insoluble
Barley	2 T dry	3.0	Insoluble
Whole wheat bread	1 slice	1.3	Insoluble
Whole wheat crackers	5 crackers	1.9	Insoluble
RyKrisp crackers	2 crackers	1.5	Insoluble
Whole wheat pasta	¼ c dry	1.9	Insoluble
Popcorn	3 c popped	3.0	Insoluble
Apple	1 small	2.8	Insoluble/soluble
Blueberries	½ c	2.5	Insoluble/soluble
Strawberries	¾ c	2.0	Insoluble/soluble
Green beans	½ c	2.3	Insoluble/soluble
Broccoli	½ c	2.0	Insoluble/soluble
Brussels sprouts	½ c	3.9	Insoluble/soluble
Spinach	½ c	2.0	Insoluble/soluble
Green peas	½ c	4.8	Insoluble/soluble

carbohydrate and low-fat diet it can often lead to improved control of diabetes with less medication in individuals with Type II diabetes mellitus.

Table 7 describes the two types of fiber. One type is the *water-insoluble* kind found in whole grains and bran. These fibers are identified as cellulose, hemicellulose, and lignins, and are indigestible. Insoluble fiber adds bulk, holds water, and moves food through the intestinal tract at a faster rate. A diet high in insoluble fiber is recommended by the American Cancer Society to reduce risk of colon cancer.

The other type of fiber is *water-soluble* fiber and includes guar, pectins, and gums. This type of fiber seems to work best in helping to control blood sugar and blood cholesterol levels. In fact, consum-

Table 8 Major Nutrients

Nutrient	Major Food Source	Body Purpose
Protein	Meat, fish, poultry, eggs, dairy products, dried peas and beans	Growth, maintains body cells, makes up part of the enzymes that control processes to keep the body functioning
Carbohydrate	Fruits, vegetables, whole grains and cereals	Provides energy
Fat	Margarine, vegetable oils, salad dressing	Provides essential fatty acids and fat-soluble vitamins A, D, E, and K, part of the structure of every cell
Calcium	Dairy products, dark green leafy vegetables	Helps give structure to bones and teeth and maintains bone health
Iron	Lean red meat, enriched cereals and grains, dried beans and peas	Involved in tissue respiration needed for the prevention of anemia
Vitamin A	Dark green vegetables, carrots, sweet potatoes	Helps maintain healthy skin, helps eyes adjust to darkness, may be important in cancer prevention
Thiamine (B_1)	Enriched cereals and grains, lean pork, nuts	Helps the nervous system function, aids in the utilization of energy
Riboflavin (B_2)	Dairy products, enriched cereals and grains	Aids in the utilization of energy
Niacin	Lean beef, poultry, fish, enriched cereals and grains	Aids in the utilization of energy; promotes healthy skin, nerves, and digestive tract

ing as little as 2 ounces of oat bran (which contains primarily soluble fiber) daily can help lower blood cholesterol levels in healthy individuals and can do so significantly when coupled with a low-cholesterol, low-fat diet. As Table 7 indicates, a person can obtain more soluble fiber by eating legumes, fruits, and vegetables as well.

Nutrient	Major Food Source	Body Purpose
Pyridoxine	Lean pork, nuts	Necessary for protein synthesis and for growth, helps fight disease
Pantothenic Acid	All plant and animal foods	Helps use energy from carbohydrates, fats, and proteins
Vitamin B_{12}	Low-fat meats, fish, poultry	Necessary for formation of red blood cells and a healthy nervous system
Vitamin C	Citrus fruits, potatoes, peppers, broccoli, tomatoes	Helps fight infection, helps in wound and bone healing
Vitamin D	Dairy products with vitamin D added	Helps build and maintain strong bones and teeth
Vitamin E	Whole grains, nuts, wheat germ	Protects red blood cells; acts as an antioxidant to prevent the destruction of vitamin A and polyunsaturated fat
Magnesium	Green leafy vegetables, whole grains, nuts	Maintains nerve and skin function
Phosphorus	Dairy products, meats, fish	Helps build and maintain strong bones and teeth, helps maintain calcium levels in blood
Potassium	Oranges, potatoes, bananas	Controls the amount of fluid in body cells
Sodium	Table salt, high-sodium condiments	Controls the amount of fluid in body cells
Zinc	All animal products, shellfish	Necessary for proper growth, wound healing
Folacin	Green leafy vegetables, beef	Necessary for formation of red blood cells

How much fiber should a person eat in one day? Current estimates indicate that dietary fiber intake of adults in the United States ranges from about 10 to 30 grams per day. The American Diabetes Association recommends a daily fiber intake of up to 40 grams. A level of maximum benefit has not been established, but levels higher than 50 grams per day may cause gastrointestinal distress and mineral malabsorption. It is best to increase your fiber intake gradually, rather than making drastic changes in your diet. Most people can safely double their fiber intake by using more of the vegetables, dried beans, and cereals listed in Table 7. Gradually try to work up to the 30- to 40-gram level, making sure that your water intake is adequate to prevent any gastrointestinal distress.

MICRONUTRIENTS: VITAMINS AND MINERALS

Vitamins and minerals, sometimes called the helper nutrients, are micronutrients, substances the body needs in exceedingly small amounts that it cannot manufacture on its own. Most are involved in regulating body processes, including skin and bone formation and blood clotting.

Each vitamin and mineral has its own functions, but they often depend on each other to be utilized most effectively. For example, vitamin D is necessary for the body to use calcium and phosphorus to build and maintain strong bones and teeth.

Table 8 lists the major vitamins and minerals, their functions, and food sources. Some foods contain a large amount of a particular vitamin or mineral (such as calcium in milk or vitamin C in citrus fruits), but, for the most part, most foods offer smaller amounts of many vitamins and minerals. No single food offers all the vitamins and minerals we need, which is why we require a variety of foods every day.

Do you need a vitamin and mineral supplement? Most vitamins and minerals have been promoted at one time or another as "cures" for various major diseases afflicting the American public. For example, vitamin C is popular as a treatment for the common cold, although we still lack definitive scientific evidence to prove that it can fulfill this role. Copper and chromium are said to help in the metabolism of glucose for people with diabetes, but once again these claims haven't been proven. There is no good reason for anyone to be taking large doses of *single* vitamins or minerals, unless a physician prescribes them for a specific medical condition, or if a certain medication alters your need for a specific vitamin or mineral. As a matter of fact, many of these substances can be toxic in large doses or may cause imbalances in other nutrients when consumed in large quantities.

Many people, however, *can* benefit greatly from taking a reasonable vitamin-mineral supplement that helps them to meet their recommended daily allowance (RDA) for nutrients, as established by the National Research Council. Those of us missing a well-rounded diet, such as some elderly people, many people on weight-loss diets, rapidly growing and developing children and adolescents, and frequent fast-food customers, need a vitamin-mineral supplement as a form of nutritional insurance. At this time, there is no scientific evidence to suggest that those with diabetes require extra amounts of any particular vitamin or mineral, unless they fall into one of these categories.

In the United States, about 1 in 4 adults has elevated blood pressure or hypertension. There are several minerals that deserve special discussion because of their relationship to hypertension. These are sodium, potassium, calcium, and magnesium.

Sodium is one of the factors known to play a role in the regulation of blood pressure, although not everyone is equally susceptible to the hazards of excess sodium in the diet. Sodium occurs naturally in some foods and is added to the diet as salt or sodium chloride. In populations with low sodium intakes, high blood pressure is rare. In contrast, in populations with high sodium intakes, high blood pressure is common. If people with high blood pressure severely restrict their sodium intakes, their blood pressure will usually fall, although not always to normal levels. Low-sodium diets may help prevent high blood pressure in susceptible individuals and help control blood pressure in those with hypertension.

The recommended sodium intake for adults is 1100 to 3300 milligrams or ½ to 1½ teaspoons of salt per day. Americans now consume an average of 2 to 4 teaspoons per day. About one third of the sodium we consume is naturally present in the foods we eat. Another third comes from using the saltshaker, and the final third comes from processed foods. For example, some of the reduced-calorie frozen dinners contain over 1000 milligrams of sodium each. One fast-food burger can contain up to 1500 milligrams of sodium, and an ounce of breakfast cereal often contains as much as 300 to 350 milligrams. The American Diabetes Association recommends an intake of 1000 milligrams of sodium per 1000 calories, or a maximum of 3000 milligrams per day. The boxes on pages 28–29 give you tips on how to reduce your intake of salt.

The ratio of sodium to potassium in a person's diet may also be an important factor in the development of hypertension. Hypertensive individuals should make an effort to increase intake of potas-

SODIUM IN YOUR DIET

The American Heart Association and the American Diabetes Association recommend that daily sodium intake not exceed 3 grams. The sodium intake for the average American is anywhere from 2400 to 7200 milligrams per day, or about 3½ teaspoons salt. Statistics show that processed foods and table salt (which is 40 percent sodium) are the major sources of sodium in our diet.

Limiting Sodium

Gradually begin lowering the sodium in your diet by following these suggestions:

1. Avoid commercially processed foods that contain large quantities of sodium — canned, smoked, salted, and pickled foods like canned soups, frozen dinners, luncheon meats, bacon, sausage, salted chips and crackers, and pickles. Opt for fresh, unprocessed foods.
2. Don't add salt to foods at the table or when cooking. Salt is an acquired taste; you can reverse your craving for sodium by limiting the amount you add to foods. Always taste your food before adding salt and gradually decrease the number of shakes.
3. Replace canned foods, such as canned vegetables, with fresh or frozen foods.
4. Avoid salty condiments and substitute low-sodium seasonings to flavor foods. High-sodium condiments include soy sauce, salty spice mixes (celery salt, garlic salt, onion salt, etc.). Low-sodium seasonings include various herbs and spices. Lemon and lime juice, fresh garlic and onions, and green peppers also enhance the flavor of foods. Try herb and spice combinations on pages 30–31.
5. Read food labels and look for ingredients that contain sodium, such as MSG, baking soda, baking powder, and sea salt. Food label terms such as "low sodium," "very low sodium," and "sodium free" mean that sodium content per serving must be 140 milligrams, 35 milligrams, and 5 milligrams or less, respectively. "Reduced sodium" means sodium content of the food is reduced by 75 percent. "Unsalted," "no salt added," "without added salt," mean that the product has not been processed with salt.
6. Avoid medications with a high sodium content, including some antacids and cough syrups.
7. Rinse canned foods, such as tuna fish and vegetables, in water to decrease the amount of sodium.

FURTHER TIPS FOR LOWERING SODIUM

Replace:	*With:*
Chips and crackers	No-Fry Tortilla Chips*
Salted pretzels	Old-Fashioned Wheat Pretzels*
Salted popcorn and salted nuts	Air-popped unsalted popcorn and unsalted dry roasted nuts or Cereal Crunch*
Canned and dehydrated soups	Homemade soups*
Bouillon cubes and canned chicken broth	Chicken Stock* or low-sodium chicken broth
Instant oatmeal	Muesli*
Ketchup	Spicy Catsup*
Canned vegetables	Italian Vegetables* or Stir-Fried Vegetables*
Olives and dill pickles	Black Forest Mushrooms* or Spinach-Stuffed Mushrooms* or fresh carrot and jicama sticks
Bottled spaghetti sauce	Marinara Sauce*
Flavored rice mix	Spanish Rice*
Biscuit and pancake mix	Basil Rolls* or French Toast Bake*

*Recipes in Part Two

sium, which is found mainly in fresh fruits and vegetables. This is particularly important if they are taking diuretics to treat hypertension which causes loss of potassium.

In population studies, calcium intake has been found to be lower in hypertensive patients than in nonhypertensive patients. Low blood levels of another mineral, magnesium, are also associated with higher blood pressure. We encourage increased intakes of foods rich in these two minerals, such as low-fat dairy products and grains.

OTHER DIETARY VARIABLES

Water Surprisingly enough, water is our most important nutrient, contributing to over half of our body weight. Although it provides no calories, every cell in our bodies depends on water to carry out essential functions. About half of our body is water. Sources of

HERB AND SPICE COMBINATIONS

Poultry and Seafood

Rosemary and thyme

Tarragon, marjoram, and onion powder, and garlic

Cumin, bay leaf, and saffron (or turmeric)

Ginger, cinnamon, and allspice

Curry powder, thyme, and onion powder

Cumin and oregano

Tarragon, thyme, parsley, and garlic

Thyme, fennel, saffron, and red pepper

Ginger, sesame seeds, and white pepper

Cilantro, parsley, cumin, and garlic

Meats

Thyme, bay leaf, and instant minced onion

Ginger, dry mustard, and garlic

Dill, nutmeg, and allspice

Black pepper, bay leaf, and cloves

Chili powder, cinnamon, and oregano

Caraway seeds, red pepper, and paprika

Thyme, dry mustard, and sage

Oregano and bay leaf

Anise, ginger, and sesame seeds

Tarragon, bay leaf, and garlic

Eggs and Cheese

Any one of the following, alone or in combination: allspice, basil, bay leaves, caraway seeds, cinnamon, cloves, ginger, marjoram, oregano, paprika, rosemary, sage, sesame seeds, thyme

Potatoes, Rice, and Pasta

Potatoes — Dill, onion powder, and parsley; caraway seeds and onion powder; nutmeg and chives, rosemary, paprika

Rice — Chili powder and cumin; curry powder, ginger, and coriander; cinnamon, cardamom, and cloves

Pasta — Basil, rosemary, and parsley; cumin, turmeric, and red pepper; oregano and thyme

water, such as milk, juice, and fruits and vegetables, are plentiful in our diets. However, we advise you to make a conscious effort to drink about eight glasses of water daily. If you are losing a great deal of water due to vomiting, diarrhea, sweating, or urinating, it is necessary to increase your fluid intake even further.

Vegetables

Asparagus — Cinnamon, paprika, basil

Beans (green) — Marjoram and rosemary; caraway seeds, thyme

Broccoli — Ginger and garlic; sesame seeds and nutmeg; thyme

Cabbage — Celery seeds and dill; curry powder and nutmeg; caraway seeds

Carrots — Cinnamon and nutmeg; ginger and onion powder; allspice; basil

Corn — Chili powder and cumin; dill and onion powder

Eggplant — Basil, oregano, sage

Peas — Anise and onion powder; rosemary and marjoram

Spinach — Curry powder and ginger; nutmeg and garlic; basil

Squash (summer) — Mint and parsley; tarragon and garlic; allspice; basil

Squash (winter) — Cinnamon and nutmeg; allspice and red pepper

Tomatoes — Basil and rosemary; oregano

Fruits

Apples — Cinnamon, allspice, and nutmeg; ginger and curry powder

Bananas — Allspice and cinnamon; nutmeg and ginger

Peaches — Coriander and mint; cinnamon and ginger

Oranges — Cinnamon and cloves

Pears — Ginger and cardamom; cinnamon

Strawberries — Cinnamon and ginger; nutmeg

Tips for Seasoning Dishes

- For best flavor, use fresh herbs. Otherwise, 1 tablespoon fresh herb = ½ teaspoon crushed dried herb.
- Increase the amount of spices and herbs by about one quarter when eliminating salt from a dish.
- To retain freshness, store dried herbs and spices in tightly sealed containers away from sunlight and heat. Replace frequently.

Alcohol The decision to include alcohol in the diet of a person with diabetes is highly individual. Your physician is the best one to tell you how much, if any, drinking is safe for you. For most people whose diabetes is diet-controlled, an occasional drink of beer, wine, or hard liquor should not be harmful. Small amounts of alcohol, *taken* *close to or during a meal,* produce little change in blood sugar levels. Alcohol itself does not raise blood glucose since the body treats it like fat, but the *carbohydrate* in beer, wine, liqueurs, and sugary mixers may cause an elevation in blood glucose. Alcohol increases the risk of hypoglycemia because it can cause blood glucose levels to drop if you have not eaten for several hours.

Diabetes pills (particularly the "first generation") and other medications may not mix with alcohol. Once again, check with your physician before imbibing.

The calories in alcoholic beverages need to be counted in your daily meal plan, particularly if you are trying to lose weight. If you take insulin or a diabetes pill, are of normal weight, and your diabetes is under control, you may be able to take an occasional drink without making substitutions in your meal plan or adjusting your medication. To prevent hypoglycemia, do *not* omit any food from your meal plan when drinking, *and do not drink on an empty stomach!*

Sweeteners The recipes in this book use a variety of sweeteners, including both calorie-containing and noncalorie-containing ones. The calorie-containing sweeteners or sugars will raise blood sugars and must be included in your meal plan. The noncalorie sweeteners will not raise blood glucose levels and will contribute few, if any, calories.

It is not harmful to ingest a small amount of table sugar, honey, molasses, maple syrup, or other sugars if they are accompanied by wholesome ingredients and nutrients and if your blood glucose is under control. In fact, the American Diabetes Association is now saying that people with diabetes can consume up to 1 teaspoon of any of these sugars per reasonable serving of food. (The maximum number of servings or teaspoons of sugar per day depends on individual caloric needs.) The largest amount per serving of any of these sugars we have used in our recipes is ¾ teaspoon. Our recipe testing has shown us that this is the smallest amount that will still render a slightly sweet flavor. We use fruit in moderation — fresh, dried, and juice — to enhance the sweet flavor of the other sugars.

The box on p. 32 lists the most commonly available caloric and noncaloric sweeteners that offer an alternative to sucrose and other sugars. There are advantages and disadvantages associated with the use of each one. The type of sweetener you choose depends on your calorie requirements, how well your diabetes is controlled, and the type of food you are consuming. Sometimes a combination of sweet-

ALTERNATIVE SWEETENERS

Caloric	Noncaloric
Fructose	Saccharin
Sugar alcohols	Cyclamate*
Sorbitol	Aspartame†
Mannitol	Acesulfame-K†

*Use currently banned in the United States
†Contributes virtually no calories when used in manufactured products; as a pourable powder it contains a minimal number of calories.

eners is appropriate and can enable you to use a lesser amount if they have a synergistic effect. It is not uncommon to find a food product that contains both types of sweeteners — caloric and noncaloric. For example, some frozen yogurts will combine aspartame and a small amount of a refined sugar to obtain a desired sweetness. You *do* need to count the calorie-containing sugars in your meal plan, so read your labels carefully. (See chapter 5 for more information on reading labels.)

Be sure to use all sweeteners in moderation. If you have questions, consult your physician or dietitian.

Fructose is a naturally occurring sweetener found in honey and fruits and contains the same number of calories as sugar. Fructose is slightly sweeter, between 1 and 1.8 times, than sugar, and causes less of an elevation in blood glucose. In fact, if diabetes is well controlled, pure crystalline fructose will not raise blood glucose levels more than an equal amount of a complex carbohydrate. However, food manufacturers do not generally use pure fructose in their products. Most will use one of the high-fructose corn syrups that contain varying amounts of fructose — either 42, 55, or 90 percent; the rest of the carbohydrate is glucose. Research has shown that foods sweetened with high-fructose corn syrup may not offer the same benefits to people with diabetes as pure fructose does. We have used pure fructose in some of our recipes to impart a special sweeter flavor and because it is less likely than some of the other calorie-containing sugars to raise blood glucose levels.

The sugar alcohols, such as sorbitol and mannitol, are also used as sweeteners in products like chewing gum. Their major drawback is that they are approximately only half as sweet as sucrose. Accomplishing a desired level of sweetness requires more of these two sugars, which means you are consuming more calories and are more likely to experience some side effects, such as minor intestinal problems.

There are distinct advantages and disadvantages associated with the use of the most common noncaloric sweeteners, cyclamates, saccharin, and aspartame. Cyclamates are currently banned from use in the U.S. The Food and Drug Administration is reviewing their safety, and they may be rereleased, perhaps by the time this book is published. Saccharin is 200 to 300 times as sweet as sucrose. It comes in liquid, powder, or tablet form. Although some people experience an unpleasant metallic aftertaste, saccharin is currently recognized as safe for use. NutraSweet, or aspartame, is a relatively new noncaloric sweetener. It is a protein that is 160 to 200 times as sweet as sucrose. It is marketed in a powdered form that uses a filler containing carbohydrates and calories. It is usually purchased in packets that each contain 4 calories. One packet has the sweetening power of 2 teaspoons of sugar. The main problem with aspartame is that it breaks down and loses its sweetness when heated and cannot be used in baked and cooked products unless added *after* cooking. It will, however, withstand microwave cooking, according to the manufacturer, provided it is not in the microwave for more than 20 minutes. You can order a free booklet, *Microwave and Cooking Recipes from NutraSweet,* from the NutraSweet Center, P.O. Box 830, Deerfield, Illinois 60015.

Acesulfame-K, or Sunette, is the newest noncaloric sweetener. It is stable to heat and can be used in baked goods. Watch for it on food labels for tabletop sweeteners, dry beverage mixes, chewing gum, and dessert and pudding mixes, alone or in combination with calorie-containing sugars. Sucralose is another new noncaloric sweetener that is currently under review by the Food and Drug Administration.

So now we have the basics under control. Let's turn next to getting something else that's very important under control — *weight*. That's the subject of our next chapter.

3

WEIGHT LOSS AND WEIGHT CONTROL

LOSING EVEN A LITTLE CAN HELP A LOT

At last count, the number of obese Americans was approaching 35 million. Due to our overabundant food supply and sedentary lifestyle, obesity in this country is not decreasing, despite the proliferation of weight-loss programs. In fact, the incidence of obesity appears still to be increasing, and a growing number of experts think many of the diets themselves are partly to blame.

A National Institutes of Health consensus conference has concluded that any level of obesity is a risk factor for several major diseases. From a medical standpoint, a body weight in excess of 20 percent above desirable weight (see Table 9) requires treatment because it is associated with a five- to sixfold increase for hypertension risk, a twofold increased risk for hypercholesterolemia, and a fourfold increased risk of Type II diabetes. And yet we can expect only a small percentage of dieters to achieve lasting success in terms of reaching their "desirable" weight, especially if they continue to use unsound, faddish diets that promise very rapid weight loss.

Fortunately, new studies show that, for many obese people, losing as little as 10 percent of body weight can help correct a tendency toward high blood pressure or diabetes. According to Dr. George Blackburn, an authority in the area of obesity research, "The whole premise that the goal of weight reduction should be to reach 'desirable' weight is the major flaw in weight-loss strategies. It's the first 10 percent of weight loss — not the last 10 percent — that's important." Modest weight losses of only 10 to 25 pounds may help counter

Table 9 How to Determine a Desirable Body Weight
1983 Metropolitan Life Height and Weight Tables

Weights are for ages 25 to 59, based on lowest mortality. They include an indoor clothing weight of 3 pounds for women and 5 pounds for men. Heights include shoes with 1-inch heels.

Men	Small Frame	Medium Frame	Large Frame	Women	Small Frame	Medium Frame	Large Frame
5'2"	128–134	131–141	138–150	4'10"	102–111	109–121	118–131
5'3"	130–136	133–143	140–153	4'11"	103–113	111–123	120–134
5'4"	132–138	135–145	142–156	5'	104–115	113–126	122–137
5'5"	134–140	137–148	144–160	5'1"	106–118	115–129	125–140
5'6"	136–142	139–151	146–164	5'2"	108–121	118–132	128–143
5'7"	138–145	142–154	149–168	5'3"	111–124	121–135	131–147
5'8"	140–148	145–157	152–172	5'4"	114–127	124–138	134–151
5'9"	142–151	148–160	155–176	5'5"	117–130	127–141	137–155
5'10"	144–154	151–163	158–180	5'6"	120–133	130–144	140–159
5'11"	146–157	154–166	161–184	5'7"	123–136	133–147	143–163
6'	149–160	157–170	164–188	5'8"	126–139	136–150	146–167
6'1"	152–164	160–174	168–192	5'9"	129–142	139–153	149–170
6'2"	155–168	164–178	172–197	5'10"	132–145	142–156	152–173
6'3"	158–172	167–182	176–202	5'11"	135–148	145–159	155–176
6'4"	162–176	171–187	181–207	6'	138–151	148–162	158–179

the major health risks associated with obesity — and these more moderate reductions in weight are much easier to maintain on a long-term basis.

ASSESSING THE RISKS: IT DEPENDS ON *WHERE* THE FAT'S AT

Research in recent years shows that obesity is no longer strictly psychological in origin. It is a complex disorder influenced by heredity, metabolism, environment, and behavior. Dr. Albert Stunkard, a psychiatrist at the University of Pennsylvania, has been able to show that adoptees resemble their biologic parents more than their adoptive parents with respect to amount and distribution of body fat. This ap-

HOW TO DETERMINE YOUR FRAME SIZE

To make an approximation of your frame size, extend your arm and bend the forearm upward at a 90-degree angle. Keep your fingers straight and turn the inside of your wrist toward the body. Place the thumb and index finger of your other hand on the two prominent bones on either side of your elbow. Measure the space between your fingers with a ruler or tape measure. Compare the number you get with the values below. These measurements are for men and women of medium frame at various heights. If your elbow measurement is less than the range given for your height, then you have a small frame. If your elbow measurement is more than the range given for your height, you have a large frame.

Men		Women	
Height in 1" Heels	*Elbow Breadth for Medium Frame*	*Height in 1" Heels*	*Elbow Breadth for Medium Frame*
5'2"–5'3"+	2½–2⅞"	4'10"–4'11"+	2¼–2½"
5'4"–5'7"+	2⅝–2⅞"	5'0"–5'3"+	2¼–2½"
5'8"–5'11"+	2¾–3"	5'4"–5'7"+	2⅜–2⅝"
6'0"–6'3"+	2¾–3⅛"	5'8"–5'11"+	2⅜–2⅝"
>6'4"	2⅞–3¼"	>6'	2½–2¾"

parent inherited tendency to be obese, with body fat predominating in specific parts of the body, is turning out to be an important determinant of risk for developing obesity-related diseases. In other words, the long-range effect of obesity on health varies from one person to another according to the amount and *location* of their fat tissue.

Some studies suggest that among patients with diabetes, *upper-body* obesity (with fat accumulating in the middle) is more prevalent than lower-body obesity (fat stored in the hips and thighs). These two types of obesity have been described as being typically "male" or apple-shaped (when fat predominates in the middle) and "female" or pear-shaped (when fat predominates in the lower half of the body). However, these two types (see Figure 1) are not always gender-specific. Many women also have upper-body obesity. Being an "apple" or "potbelly" type puts one at much higher risk for developing heart disease, high blood pressure, and diabetes than simply being overweight or a "pear," i.e., carrying weight in the lower half of the body. The reason for this may be that abdominal fat is more metabolically

Figure 1 Pear vs. Apple

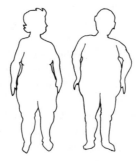

active, possibly causing abnormalities in the function of glucose, insulin, and sodium in the body. Of course, *any* form of obesity increases health risks.

It is extremely important to acknowledge and treat obesity in both men and women. Women are, typically, more likely to be concerned about their weight — for cosmetic reasons — than men. Both women *and* men should be concerned — for health reasons — particularly if they have apple-type body shapes.

AVOIDING THE YO-YO SYNDROME

Being overweight or obese is the result of energy imbalance. This means that more calories are taken into the body than are used up; unused calories are stored as excess fat. Calorie intake occurs in only *one* way — by eating. Calorie expenditure can occur in *two* ways: by fueling the body for basic metabolic needs, such as building new cells and maintaining organs, and by powering muscles to do work (walking, running, typing, etc.). It is only when calorie intake exceeds expenditure that our bodies store the excess as fat. Scientific research is trying to determine just how intricate and interrelated our body systems and environmental factors are in controlling energy intake and expenditure. What we know for certain is that "miracle cures" and quick weight-loss regimens are *not* the answer to successful *long-term* weight maintenance.

For most people, the challenge is not in *losing* weight, but in *maintaining* permanent weight loss. Millions of Americans have been caught up in the "yo-yo syndrome" — losing weight, gaining it back, losing again, and then regaining those unwanted pounds for a second or third time. Many dieters end up at an even higher weight than where they began once they have gone off their weight-loss programs. Losing weight by consuming very low calorie diets appears to increase the efficiency with which the body uses calories for fuel, so that people gain weight more easily when they go "off the wagon." In turn, it is more difficult to lose weight the second time around because of the body's new fuel efficiency. If weight loss is rapid in the beginning, the dieter loses lean body mass in addition to fat, making each further attempt at weight loss increasingly more difficult because fat tissue requires fewer calories to function than does lean tissue.

WHAT REALLY WORKS?

Anyone who is willing to make a *lifetime* commitment to improve eating and exercise habits can succeed at long-term weight loss. Most successful long-term weight-loss programs incorporate several components: behavior modification; exercise; social support; nutrition basics; and cognitive change, including goal setting, assertiveness training, and coping with mistakes and motivation. Emphasis is placed on slow, progressive weight loss.

To be truly effective, therapy for weight loss should be tailored to the needs of the individual. Some patients benefit most from basic information about diabetes and nutrition, meal planning, dining out, food labeling, etc. Oftentimes, bad habits need to be changed, including eating too many calorically dense foods, eating too much and too frequently, or binge eating. Simply keeping track of amounts eaten and timing of meals in the form of a daily food record can be very revealing and a good way to start making changes. Those who say "I hardly eat anything" may find that they are eating small quantities but are choosing very high calorie foods and are snacking frequently.

Behavioral eating problems are the most challenging and take the longest to change. Strategies for change include eliminating the "wrong" foods from the cupboard, eating only at the table at predetermined times, and developing activities and rewards not related to food. See pages 40–41 for some other weight-loss tips.

WHAT TYPE OF DIET IS MOST EFFECTIVE?

What's the best type of diet to follow for optimal weight loss? Is the same diet the best for *maintaining* weight loss? Will you need to

WEIGHT-LOSS TIPS

We all have habits that need changing if we want to accomplish permanent weight loss. Here is a list of ideas that should help you lose weight initially and then maintain your new shape:

1. Keep a food record — record the time, place, amount, and type of food you eat daily. Patterns of overeating and snacking will become obvious. Also, if you have to write it down, you may not eat it in the first place.
2. Never go shopping at the supermarket when you are hungry. You are at much higher risk of impulsively buying the wrong foods. It is best to have a shopping list and stick to it.
3. Use smaller plates and dishes — research has shown that we perceive our portion sizes relative to the size of the serving dish. Smaller plates make portions look bigger and in turn make you feel fuller after eating.
4. Restrict meals to one location. This rule will help to reduce the amount of food you eat without even thinking about it and will make you more aware of portions you are consuming.
5. Keep serving dishes in the kitchen — you will be less likely to help yourself to second portions because the food will be out of sight.
6. Put away leftovers before you start eating — save them for lunch the next day or freeze them for another meal. Store them in covered bowls and containers; if they're visible when you open the refrigerator, you will be more likely to snack on them.

spend the rest of your life eating grapefruit, counting calories and carbohydrates, and avoiding all your favorite treats and indulgences?

Our bodies are made of lean tissue (muscle, bone, water, organs) and fat mass. As we have noted, you want to lose weight in the form of fat mass and not lean muscle mass. Figure 2 (page 42) shows the percentage of weight lost as lean and fat mass on different types of weight-loss diets. For example, on the high-protein, low-carbohydrate ketogenic diets that were popular for many years, initial weight loss is primarily in the form of water and lean mass. Taking weight off quickly can be exciting, but it's less than desirable from a medical standpoint and it sets you up to quickly gain the weight back — and then some. You want a diet that really cuts into the fat, not the lean.

7. Eat before a social function where there will be food — take the edge off your hunger before entering a social setting where you will be tempted to eat high-calorie foods.

8. *Never* skip a meal — this rule is very important if you take insulin. And if you skip meals, you are often so hungry that you overeat at the next meal.

9. Set realistic goals for the amount of weight you want to lose and the amount of time you will take — don't try to lose 15 pounds in 2 weeks in order to fit into a favorite party dress.

10. Find nonfood rewards and treats — reward your success with a new outfit, a new book, a minivacation, or something else special.

11. Become more active — participating in a moderate exercise program is ideal; but don't forget that you can benefit from becoming generally more active — use stairs when possible, park a little farther away and walk, keep moving!

12. Don't weigh yourself too often — it's sometimes disappointing when your weight doesn't change as much as you would expect. Hang in there — if you're eating less you will see results!

13. Make sure you get the support you need to lose weight — family, friends, support groups, will help you continue to succeed.

14. Positive "self-talk" is great for your self-esteem and weight. Remind yourself about your good traits, the terrific changes that you are making, and the positive effects on your health and appearance.

15. Indulge yourself with habits that make you feel special and important . . . soaking in a bubble bath, calling a friend long-distance, or enjoying an occasional breakfast in bed.

The best diet for weight loss is one that you can live with permanently and that allows you to lose weight — slowly — primarily in the form of fat. Researchers at the Oregon Health Sciences University have found that the diet program that promotes maximum weight loss in the form of fat is made up of a wide variety of foods and provides 800 to 1200 calories for women and 1200 to 2000 calories for men. Adding an exercise component to the program helps to conserve lean body mass and promote overall fitness.

The most successful weight-loss programs now use a low-fat, high-carbohydrate diet similar to the recommendations of the American Diabetes Association. This type of diet is ideal for weight loss because it is less calorically dense and is greater in bulk than some

Figure 2 Percent of Weight Lost on Various Reducing Programs

■ Percent of weight loss that is lean body mass
▧ Percent of weight lost that is fat mass

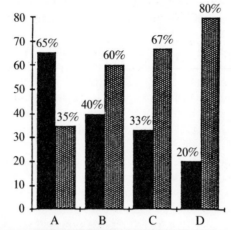

A. Starvation and low-carbohydrate ketogenic diets
B. Mixed food diets, 800–1000 calories
C. Mixed food diets, 1000–1800 calories
D. Mixed food diets, 1000–1800 calories plus mild to moderate physical activity

higher-fat diets. You get to eat a larger quantity of food for the same number of calories. You can heap your plate high! Most important, it is a style of eating that you *can,* and should, stick with for the rest of your life. Table 10 outlines two sample weight-loss plans based on the American Diabetes Association's nutritional recommendations and exchange lists. Sample menus for these plans include a number of our recipes.

Accompanied by a program of moderate exercise (see chapter 6), either a 1200-calorie plan (for women) or an 1800-calorie plan (for men) provides a sensible, safe way to lose weight and to keep it off. The recipes in this book will fit well into this weight-loss plan. Include them in your diet according to the assigned exchanges. (See chapter 5 for information on meal planning and food exchanges.)

Good luck, and remember that losing even a few pounds can be of great benefit in terms of improved glucose control. If you have Type II diabetes, trimming back your weight even moderately may enable you to avoid insulin or diabetes pills. Your doctor will determine what, if any, medication you need as your diet progresses.

Table 10   Low-Calorie Menu Plans

1200-CALORIE WEIGHT-LOSS PLAN

55% carbohydrate (165 grams)
20% protein   (60 grams)
25% fat   (33 grams)

Exchange Group	Number of Servings	Protein (grams)	Fat (grams)	Carbohydrate (grams)
Skim milk	2	16	–	24
Fruit	4	–	–	60
Vegetable	2	4	–	10
Bread/starch	5	15	–	75
Lean meat	4	28	12	–
Fat	4	–	20	–
Total		63	32	169

SAMPLE MENU

Breakfast

1 c plain nonfat yogurt topped with	1 skim milk
1¼ c sliced strawberries	1 fruit
1 Apple Oatmeal Muffin* with	1 starch/bread, ½ fat
½ t margarine	½ fat
1 vitamin and mineral supplement	
Coffee, tea, or water	

Lunch

Tuna Curry Sandwich*	1 lean meat, 1 fruit
	1 starch/bread, ½ fat
1 oz skim milk cheese	1 lean meat
½ c Sunny Salad* topped with	1 vegetable, ½ fat
2 T Low-Fat Thousand Island Dressing*	1 fat
1 small apple	1 fruit
8–10 No-Fry Tortilla Chips*	1 bread
Coffee, tea, water, or other noncaloric beverage	

Dinner

½ Chicken Breast Dijon*	2 lean meat
½ c Italian Vegetables*	1 vegetable
½ c Easy Bulgur Pilaf*	1 starch/bread, 1 fat
½ c Low-Calorie Chocolate Pudding*	1 skim milk, 1 fat
½ c Melon with Slivered Almonds and Ginger*	1 fruit
Coffee, tea, water, or other noncaloric beverage	

Snack

3 c air-popped popcorn	1 starch/bread

*Recipes in Part Two

1800-CALORIE WEIGHT-LOSS PLAN

55% carbohydrate (248 grams)
20% protein   (90 grams)
25% fat   (50 grams)

Exchange Group	Number of Servings	Protein (grams)	Fat (grams)	Carbohydrate (grams)
Skim milk	2	16	–	24
Fruit	4	–	–	60
Vegetable	3	6	–	15
Starch/bread	10	30	–	150
Lean meat	5	35	15	–
Fat	7	–	35	–
Total		87	50	249

SAMPLE MENU

Breakfast

1 c bran cereal	2 starch/bread
1 c skim milk	1 skim milk
½ banana	1 fruit
2 slices wheat toast	2 bread/starch
Dietetic jelly	free
2 t margarine	2 fat
1 vitamin and mineral supplement	
Coffee, tea, or water	

Lunch

Turkey Club Sandwich*	3 starch/bread, 2 lean meat, 1 vegetable, 2 fat
1 c Fruit Medley*	2 fruit
Coffee, tea, or water	

Dinner

3 oz Grilled Onion Burger*	3 lean meat
1 whole grain herb bun	2 starch/bread
1 T reduced-calorie mayonnaise	1 fat
1 T ketchup, mustard, dill pickle relish	free
1 c spinach salad with mushrooms, tomato, and sprouts	2 vegetables
½ T Traditional Vinaigrette Dressing*	1 fat
1¼ Strawberry Dippers*	1 fruit
Coffee, tea, or water	

*Recipes in Part Two

Snack

½ c Low-Calorie Chocolate Pudding* ......   1 skim milk, 1 fat

6 vanilla wafers ....   1 starch/bread

---

*Recipes in Part Two

4

DINING OUT AND SPECIAL OCCASIONS

DINING OUT or entertaining friends is something that we all look forward to as a relaxing and enjoyable variation on the daily routine. Diabetes need not keep you or your family from enjoying these pleasures. With the proper knowledge, you can still dine out, entertain company, and be entertained.

Of course, dining out often means adjusting other meals and snacks for the day as you plan ahead for your special meal. For example, if you know you will be eating a late dinner, have your evening snack at your usual dinner time and the larger meal at the after-dinner snack time. You can also adjust your medication accordingly if you take insulin —that is, you can take more short-acting insulin before a big meal or delay an injection if your meal time is delayed. A third option used by some people who have diabetes is to increase the amount or duration of exercise or activity for the day to allow for increased food intake. However, none of these changes in schedule should be made without obtaining a premeal blood sugar level or without the approval of your physician.

Eating out in restaurants usually results in a higher intake of fat, sugar, and calories than most of us would consume at home. It is a good idea to save your fat exchanges (see next chapter for information on food exchanges) for your meal out. The carbohydrates in the fruit exchanges in your meal plan can be substituted for sugar in sauces, gravies, and condiments. In fact, milk, fruit, and bread exchanges are similar enough in their carbohydrate content that they can be substituted fairly easily for a special meal. Keep your portion sizes close to what your food plan allows.

HOW TO REDUCE FAT IN RESTAURANT MEALS

1. Request that salad dressings, butter, margarine, mayonnaise, and sour cream be served separately on a side dish. Use lemon juice or vinegar for a dressing or bring your own low-calorie dressing from home.
2. Order clear soups, like broths or consommé, or vegetable-based soups (gazpacho) instead of cream soups.
3. Specify that no fat should be added to whatever type of chicken, fish, or red meat that you order.
4. Ask that your sandwiches be served without mayonnaise or margarine on the bread. Chicken, turkey, low-fat cheeses, and lean meats are recommended fillings.
5. Remove all visible fat from any cuts of poultry or meat.
6. Try to avoid bean salads, tuna salads, chicken salads, pasta salads, and potato salads made with mayonnaise. Choose a lettuce salad, plain vegetables, or sliced tomatoes.
7. Choose vegetables made without sauce or without added butter or margarine.
8. Avoid rich muffins, sweet rolls, and breads. Choose plain breads or rolls and low-fat crackers such as soda crackers, rye crackers, or melba toast. Use margarine or butter sparingly.

Be an inquisitive diner. Ask your waiter how a dish is prepared. Is it broiled, baked, fried, braised, breaded, or roasted? Was additional fat used in the preparation? Does the entree or side dish come with sauce, gravy, or sour cream? And don't forget to ask if the restaurant can provide you with margarine instead of butter, and low-fat or nonfat milk rather than whole. The box above offers other tips for eating out and ideas for reducing your fat intake while dining.

Eating lean in your typical American restaurant or cafeteria these days is a challenge. For example, choosing the salad bar doesn't guarantee you a low-fat meal. Add the wrong "goodies" and you can wind up with a meal that has more fat and calories than your favorite fast-food burger. High-fat, high-calorie offenders include marinated mushrooms (170 calories for 4); Cheddar cheese (57 calories per tablespoon); croutons (76 calories for 8); sunflower seeds (79 calories per tablespoon); and salads such as three-bean (85 calories per ⅓ cup), macaroni (101 calories per ⅓ cup), and carrot-raisin (115 calories per ⅓ cup). The box on p. 48 shows you how to choose your salad ingredients and dressings wisely.

PREFERRED SALAD BAR CHOICES

Alfalfa sprouts	Green and red peppers
Cucumber	Radishes
Tomato	Snow peas
Spinach	Zucchini
Carrot	Garbanzo beans
Mushrooms	Water-packed tuna
Broccoli	Boiled shrimp
Cauliflower	Plain kidney beans
Cabbage	Hard-cooked egg whites
Jicama	(skip the yolk)
Water chestnuts	Low-fat cottage cheese

Use this list to help you compare salad dressing calories:

Dressing	Calories per Tablespoon
Red wine vinegar	2
Lemon juice	4
Low-calorie blue cheese	11
Low-calorie Italian	16
Low-calorie French	22
Low-calorie Thousand Island	24
Creamy Italian	52
Ranch	54
Thousand Island	59
French	67
Italian	69
Blue cheese	77

CHOOSE A RESTAURANT THAT FEATURES WHAT YOU WANT

Consumer demand seems to be changing so that more and more Americans are requesting low-fat, low-sugar, low-calorie cuisine. And as our taste buds become more sophisticated we come to expect more than the traditional "dieter's" plate of cottage cheese, a hamburger patty, melba toast, and sliced tomatoes. In San Diego we have a growing number of restaurants that serve healthful lean cuisine that everyone can enjoy. "TrimLine" dishes, low in cholesterol, fat, sodium, and calories, and reduced in sugar, are featured on the menu at Café Lautrec in La Jolla. As you can see in the box on p. 50, the gourmet menu is international and incorporates some of the latest cooking trends. The famous Hotel del Coronado near San Diego also has two restaurants that offer light entrees on the lunch menu. For under 300 calories you can choose pasta primavera with fresh vegetables in a basil-yogurt sauce or a tomato rose stuffed with albacore. Shop around; you're likely to find similar restaurants in your own area.

EATING IN ETHNIC RESTAURANTS

Many of us enjoy eating a variety of ethnic cuisines in restaurants. Generally speaking, your best bet is to avoid the fried foods and order entrees in which meat is used as a condiment and not as a main course. Such dishes still have a full, meaty flavor but are primarily vegetables and complex carbohydrates. Preferable choices in a Mexican restaurant include corn tortillas, frijoles cocidos (boiled beans), salsa (tomato-chili sauce), carne asada (baked or broiled beef), arroz con pollo (rice with chicken), or fish Veracruz (in a fresh tomato-herb sauce).

Chinese restaurants offer many low-fat, low-cholesterol menu choices. But watch out for dishes that are "deep-fried," "dipped in batter," "sweet and sour," "in a plum sauce," or that contain peanuts and cashews. The best choices include hot and sour soup, wonton soup, stir-fried vegetables, chow mein, chop suey (lots of vegetables), Szechuan-style bean curd, and steamed rice.

Italian food also offers many healthful choices for diners. Olive oil is the preferred cooking oil, and we now know that it is good for heart health. Skip the rich cream sauces and choose pastas topped with marinara sauce or tossed in olive oil. Meatless spinach lasagna, chicken cacciatore, and vegetable pizzas using skim-milk mozzarella are good choices. Contact your local affiliate of the American Diabetes Association for more detailed information on the nutrient composition and exchange values of different ethnic meals, typical of those available in area restaurants.

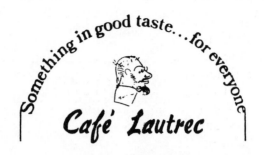

Something in good taste...for everyone

Café Lautrec

SPECIAL "TRIMLINE" CUISINE FROM CAFÉ LAUTREC IN LA JOLLA, CALIFORNIA

Low-calorie, Low-cholesterol, Low-sodium

Soups:

Icy Spicy Gazpacho

Vegetable Supreme

Chicken Florentine

Fresh Fish Chowder

Salads:

Chicken Mandarin

Skinny Minnie

TrimLine Toastada

Entrees:

Thai Peanut Chicken

Chicken Breast Stuffed with Apples and Almonds

Turkey Burger

Hungarian Goulash

Greek Lamb Avgolemono

Lamb Curry

Swordfish Brochette with Brown and Wild Rice

Shrimp Creole

Fresh Linguini with:

Artichokes and Feta

Red Pepper Pesto

Scallops and Snow Peas

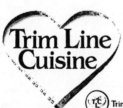

Trim Line Cuisine

Trim Line Cuisine: Low calorie, low cholesterol, low sodium

FAST FOODS

Fast-food restaurants are a way of life in the United States. From 1970 to 1980, the number of fast-food restaurants increased from 30,000 to 140,000. Fast-food sales represent 2 dollars out of every 5 spent in restaurants these days. The main advantage to this type of food is that it is fast, easy, and convenient. One nutritional advantage is that the meals are high in protein, but there are many disadvantages, too, unless one chooses wisely. In general, fast foods are too high in calories, fat, saturated fat, sodium, and sugar and too low in fiber.

Increasing consumer awareness and demand for more healthful food choices is bringing about some changes in the fast-food industry. Many restaurants now feature salad bars or salad selections with "lite" or dietetic dressings. Charbroiled food items are becoming popular. Carl's Jr. has a charbroiled chicken sandwich that is approved by the American Heart Association. Other restaurants have added baked potatoes to the menu, a good choice if the topping is low in calories and fat. Sugar-free soft drinks and low-fat milk are widely available as well. Be sure to order the smaller portions and avoid deluxe, double, or "whopper" styles.

Fortunately, many fast-food restaurants are also making an effort to reduce the sodium content of their meals. Table 11 provides you with information on the nutrient content of different fast foods as of late 1989. As you can see, one hamburger or cheeseburger can contain between 1 gram and 1.8 grams of sodium. Remember, the American Diabetes Association's recommended sodium intake is 2 to 3 grams for the entire day!

Be aware of what you are eating when you choose a fast-food meal. Approximately how many calories and how much fat, sugar, and salt does the meal contain? How do these values fit into your meal plan for the day? Balance your food choices for the rest of the day accordingly, and an occasional trip to a fast-food restaurant will not undermine an otherwise healthful diet.

CELEBRATIONS AND SPECIAL OCCASIONS

Holidays, birthdays, anniversaries, and other special occasions are a time to celebrate with good friends, good will, and good food. The menus and recipes in the special occasions chapter of Part Two are included to give you ideas on how to prepare healthful, good-

Table 11 Fast-Food Facts

Food	Serving	Calories	Protein (grams)	Fat (grams)	Percent Calories from Fat (%)	Carbo-hydrate (grams)	Sodium (mg)	Exchanges
Burger King Whopper with cheese	1	711	31	43	54	47	1164*	3 starch/bread, 3 medium-fat meat, 6 fat
Jack in the Box Cheese Nachos	1	570	15	35	55	49	1154*	3 starch/bread, 1 medium-fat meat, 6 fat
Jack in the Box Supreme Crescent	1	547	20	40	66	27	1053*	2 starch/bread, 2 medium-fat meat, 6 fat
Kentucky Fried Chicken Original Recipe	half breast	276	20	17	54	10	654*	½ starch/bread, 3 medium-fat meat
McDonald's Big Mac	1	563	26	33	53	41	1010*	2½ starch/bread, 3 medium-fat meat, 3 fat
McDonald's Chicken McNuggets	1	323	19	20	56	15	512	1 starch/bread, 2 medium-fat meat, 2 fat

Food	Serving	Calories	Protein (grams)	Fat (grams)	Percent Calories from Fat (%)	Carbo-hydrate (grams)	Sodium (mg)	Exchanges
McDonald's fries	regular	220	3	12	49	26	109	2 starch/bread, 2 fat
Taco Bell Burrito Supreme	1	457	21	22	43	43	952*	3 starch/bread, 2 medium-fat meat, 2 fat
Wendy's bacon-and-cheese potato	1	570	19	30	47	57	1180*	3½ starch/bread, 1 medium-fat meat, 5 fat
Wendy's fish fillet	3 oz	210	14	11	47	13	475	1 starch/bread, 2 medium-fat meat
Wendy's garden salad: lettuce, egg, cheese, potato salad, ham, 2 T Italian dressing	~4 cups	~ 470	20	23	44	27	1131*	1 starch/bread, 2 medium-fat meat, 1 lean meat, 1 vegetable, 4 fat
Wendy's Triple Cheeseburger	1	1040	72	68	59	35	1848*	2½ starch/bread, 9 medium-fat meat, 4 fat

Healthy Choices: either low in fat or contains fat that is not highly saturated

Food	Serving	Calories	Protein (grams)	Fat (grams)	Percent Calories from Fat (%)	Carbo-hydrate (grams)	Sodium (mg)	Exchanges
Carl's Jr. char-broiled chicken sandwich	1	320	28	9	25	30	n.a.	3 lean meat, 2 starch/bread
Domino's Cheese Pizza	2 slices of 12"	340	18	6	16	52	660*	3 starch/bread, 1 medium-fat meat, 1 vegetable
Jack in the Box Chicken Fajita Pita	1	292	24	8	25	29	703*	2½ lean meat, 2 starch/bread
McDonald's shrimp salad	1	102	14	3	26	5	571	1½ lean meat, 1 vegetable
Pollo Loco Roasted Chicken	4 oz (⅓ c rice and chicken plus ¼ c pinto beans)	410	34	14	31	30	n.a.	4 lean meat, 2 starch/bread
Roy Rogers roast beef sandwich	regular	317	27	10	28	29	785*	2 starch/bread, 3 lean meat

Food	Serving	Calories	Protein (grams)	Fat (grams)	Percent Calories from Fat (%)	Carbo-hydrate (grams)	Sodium (mg)	Exchanges
Shakey's thin crust vegetable (mushroom, onion, green pepper) cheese pizza	1/10 of 13"	171	10	5	26	21	395	1 starch/bread, 1 medium-fat meat, 1 vegetable
Taco Bell Tostado	1	179	9	6	30	25	101	1½ starch/bread, 1 medium-fat meat
Wendy's Chicken Breast Fillet on Bun	1	320	25	10	28	31	500	2 starch/bread, 3 lean meat
Wendy's garden salad: lettuce, pasta salad, raisins, sunflower seeds, 2 T reduced-calorie dressing	~4 cups	~ 340	29	8	21	21	400	1 starch/bread, 1 high-fat meat, 1 vegetable, ½ fruit, 2 fat
Wendy's plain baked potato	1	250	6	2	3	52	60	3½ starch/bread

*High in sodium (>600 mg). Monitor intake.

tasting cuisine for your family and friends. Most of these recipes call for more fat than the recommended daily intake, which is why you should reserve them for special events. However, we ask you to use either a monounsaturated or polyunsaturated fat or oil, keeping saturated or animal fat to a minimum. And always trim the higher-fat cuts of meat, such as lamb and pork. As you would when dining out, plan ahead to save calories and fat exchanges for your special meal.

If you like to cook with wine, you should be aware of recently released information from the U.S. Department of Agriculture. It has always been thought that most of the alcohol in hot dishes evaporates during the cooking process, enhancing the flavor of the food but adding very few extra calories. The new research shows, however, that the amount of alcohol a dish retains depends on how it is prepared and the length of time it is cooked or baked. See Table 12 for specific guidelines.

ALCOHOL

Each of the recipes in the special occasions chapter is accompanied by an optional wine selection. Refer to chapter 2 for general

Table 12   Cooking with Wine

Preparation	Percent of Alcohol Retained
Immediate consumption, without heat	100
Overnight storage, without heat	70
Boiling liquid with added alcohol, removed from heat	85
Flamed	75
Baked, approximately 25 minutes, alcohol not stirred into mixture	45
Baked or simmered, alcohol stirred into mixture:	
15 minutes	40
30 minutes	35
1 hour	25
1½ hours	20
2 hours	10
2½ hours	5

Source: United States Department of Agriculture, Agricultural Research Service, 1989

considerations regarding the use of alcohol in the diabetic diet. If you do consume alcohol, you should do so in moderation — no more than 1 to 2 alcohol "equivalents," once or twice a week. One equivalent is equal to the amount of alcohol in:

- a 1½-ounce shot of distilled beverage (gin, rum, Scotch, vodka, whiskey, dry brandy)
- 4 ounces of dry wine
- 12 ounces of beer

Alcohol contains 7 calories per gram and is metabolized by the body in a manner similar to fat. It is best to substitute it for fat exchanges in your diet. One equivalent is equal to 90 calories or 2 fat exchanges.

If you do decide to have a drink with your special meal, one of the best choices you can make is a *dry* wine, such as the ones we recommend in Part Two. These wines are all moderately priced and are available in most areas.

5 ═══════════════

MEAL PLANNING, FOOD EXCHANGES, AND LONG-TERM MANAGEMENT

Successful long-term management of diabetes requires attention to meal planning. We will explain the basic exchange system for planning diabetic diets in this chapter. Additional approaches to meal planning include basic nutrition guidelines, individualized menus, calorie counting, and a simple one-page tool from the American Diabetes Association, entitled "Healthy Food Choices." Choosing the right meal plan depends on your own nutritional, social, and medical needs. A combination of meal planning tools is often useful as these needs change over time. The emphasis now is on flexibility and creativity in using different meal planning approaches for the management of diabetes.

Meal planning should not be considered a "diet," but rather a "realistic way to eat." Remember, a meal plan should enable a person to accomplish the following nutritional goals:

- good overall nutrition
- maintenance of desirable weight or weight loss
- acceptable blood sugar levels
- acceptable blood fat levels

It is important that each diabetic seek the assistance of a qualified health professional, that is, a Registered Dietitian and member of the American Dietetic Association, when it comes time to plan a diet that meets individual needs. The information in this chapter will help you implement what you learn from a dietitian and will help you maintain a proper diet for life.

EXCHANGE LISTS FOR MEAL PLANNING

What is the exchange system for meal planning? This system groups foods into *six lists* called *exchange lists*. Each list is made up of a group of measured foods of approximately the same nutritional value, so that they can be substituted, or exchanged, with other foods in the same list. One exchange is approximately equal to another in the same group in terms of calories, carbohydrates, protein, and fat.

The exchange system offers more structure and in-depth information about diet. Meal planning based on the number and types of exchanges appropriate for the patient or client is highly individual. The system is a valuable tool to help clients learn about basic nutrition and nutrient and calorie content of foods. A copy of the exchange lists begins on p. 338.

MENU APPROACHES TO MEAL PLANNING

Whether you want a short- or long-term dietary management plan, individualized menus that contain specific foods and portion sizes designed to meet a specific nutrient prescription can be the answer. It is important to seek out the qualified guidance of a Registered Dietitian to help you in your menu planning, rather than rely on the standardized, preprinted plans that are widely available. The Registered Dietitian can tailor menus to your needs, which is what really contributes to long-term dietary success.

COUNTING APPROACHES FOR MEAL PLANNING

Calorie counting is a popular and successful method for losing weight; it can also be helpful in planning a diabetic diet. It is most appropriate for those who are overweight and have non-insulin-dependent diabetes. Generally, with this approach, a calorie level is established by the dietitian based on individual need, and allows for a 1- to 2-pound weight loss per week. The patient makes food choices based on lists or reference books that provide calorie content of foods. Keeping a record of food and calorie intake is essential for success.

Other counting approaches to meal planning include the point system (to count carbohydrates) and something called the "total available glucose" (TAG) approach. Both of these require more detailed explanation and instruction by a dietitian, but they offer more flexibility to meet the individual needs of people with diabetes and their families.

SICK DAYS

When you have a fever, the flu, an infection, or other illness, diabetes can quickly get out of control. The body releases hormones in response to the stress of illness. These hormones also raise blood glucose levels, increasing the body's need for more insulin. If you are taking insulin you must continue to take it during the illness to prevent increasingly high blood glucose levels. If you take oral hypoglycemics or diabetes pills, continue to take them as well, except during periods of vomiting.

It is best to develop a sick-day management plan with your physician *before* you become ill. Include enough liquid and calories from carbohydrate to prevent hypoglycemia and dehydration. The exchanges which contain carbohydrate are milk, vegetables, fruits, and breads. If your body is not tolerating regular foods well, replace carbohydrates in the meal plan with liquid, semi-liquid, or soft foods. In this case, the source of carbohydrate (including sugar-containing liquids) is not of major concern. Also be sure to consume 8 to 12 ounces of fluid every hour. If the illness lasts for more than 24 hours or if vomiting and diarrhea persist for more than a few hours, be sure to contact your physician.

CHOOSING THE RIGHT FOODS: HOW TO READ
A FOOD LABEL

After you and your doctor have decided on the right meal plan, the next step is to learn to choose the right foods. How do you translate the meal pattern into your daily diet? To choose the right foods, you will need to learn to read food labels for ingredients and nutrition information. Ingredient labels appear on just about every packaged food product. Reading the ingredient list of a food product will tell you two important things — the relative amounts of each ingredient and whether the product contains some type of sugar.

Ingredients are listed by weight in descending order of predominance. Therefore, the ingredient that is present in the largest amount is listed first, and so on down the line. If sugar is one of the first three ingredients listed for a food, then it is probably present in a fairly significant amount. If it is the fourth or fifth ingredient, then the amount of sugar is much less and probably not significant.

Another important thing the ingredients list tells you is the type of sugar, if any, contained in the product. These sugar types include:

brown sugar	glucose	levulose	sorbitol
corn syrup	honey	mannitol	sucrose
dextrose	invert sugar	maple syrup	xylitol
fructose	lactose	molasses	

Generally, words that end in "ose" or "ol" are some form of sugar. Some products contain a combination of the various sweeteners listed here. If they are added together, they can account for a significant proportion of the food, so beware.

The phrases "nutritive sweetener" and "non-nutritive sweetener" are often used on food products. A nutritive sweetener is one that contains calories, such as the sugars we have listed. The term non-nutritive sweetener identifies a sweetener that contains very few or no calories, such as aspartame (trade name NutraSweet or Equal) and saccharin. More and more often non-calorie-containing sweeteners are combined with the various types of calorie-containing sugars in foods. Read the product label carefully to determine how this type of food fits into your meal plan. Table 13 lists the nutrient content and suggested exchange values for some frozen desserts that are available at your supermarket. As you can see, some contain as many as five or six different types of sweeteners — both caloric and noncaloric. So, even products that boast noncaloric sweeteners in their advertisements may contain calories and carbohydrates from other added sugars. Learn to be a savvy consumer and a dedicated label reader!

An ingredients list will alert you to two other items to monitor in your diet — the type of fat and the amount of salt. Be particularly careful to watch for fats that are highly saturated. These include most fat from animal sources, such as bacon, beef, butter, and lard; and three fats from the vegetable kingdom: coconut, cocoa butter (chocolate), and palm oil. It is important to remember that a label can list palm or coconut oil as "vegetable oil" or "vegetable fat," so that you cannot be sure that you are consuming a beneficial fat when you see this generic term. Appropriate fats to look for in processed foods include corn, safflower, sesame, and sunflower oils, soybean oil (partially hydrogenated), and cottonseed oil. High-sodium ingredients, in addition to salt, include baking powder, baking soda, monosodium glutamate, soy sauce, and bouillon.

Table 13 The Different Sweeteners Used in Frozen Desserts and Bars

Product	Sweeteners Used	Calories (per serving)	Carbohydrate (grams)	Fat (grams)	Protein (grams)	Exchange Information
Sugar-Free Popsicle Ice Pops	Fruit juice, aspartame	18	5	0	0	free
Sugar-Free Fudgesicle Fudge Pops	Maltodextrin, aspartame	35	6	1	2	½ starch/bread
Crystal Light Bars	Fruit juice, aspartame	14	2	0	0	free
Crystal Light Cool 'n Creamy Frozen Bavarian Bars Orange/Vanilla	Fruit juice, corn syrup, high-fructose corn syrup, aspartame, maltodextrin	30	5	1	1	½ fruit
Crystal Light Cool 'n Creamy Frozen Bavarian Bars	Corn syrup, aspartame	50	7	2	2	½ low-fat milk or ½ starch/bread
Carnation Creamy Lites Frozen Snack Bars	Polydextrose, sugar, aspartame	50	5	2	2	½ low-fat milk or ½ starch/bread
Weight Watchers Chocolate Mousse	Polydextrose, sorbitol, aspartame	35	9	<1	2	½ starch/bread
Weight Watchers Vanilla Sandwich Bar	Sugar, corn syrup, dextrose	150	28	3	3	1 starch/bread 1 fruit
Weight Watchers Double Fudge Frozen Dessert	Sugar	60	12	1	3	1 starch/bread
Weight Watchers Orange/Vanilla Treat	Sugar, corn syrup	60	12	1	3	1 starch/bread
Sugar-Free Eskimo Pie	Sorbitol, polydextrose, aspartame, mannitol	140	11	12	3	1 starch/bread 2 Fat

Product	Sweeteners Used	Calories (per serving)	Carbohydrate (grams)	Fat (grams)	Protein (grams)	Exchange Information
Yoplait Soft Frozen Yogurt	Corn syrup, fruit purée, corn syrup solids, sugar	90	15	3	2	1 starch/bread
Knudsen Pushups Lowfat Frozen Yogurt	Sugar, corn syrup, fruit or fruit purée	90	19	1	1	1½ fruit
Dannon Frozen Yogurt on a Stick	Sugar, corn sweetener, fruit, fruit purée	50	8	1	2	½ low-fat milk or ½ starch/bread
Shamitoff's Fruit and Cream Bars	Fruit, sugar, corn sweetener	85	16	2	1	1 starch/bread
Welch's Fruit Juice Bars	Fruit juice, sugar, fruit purée	45	11	0	0	1 fruit
Dole Fruit 'n Juice Bars	Fruit, fruit juice, sugar, corn sweetener, corn syrup	70	17	<1	<1	1 fruit
Dole Fruit and Cream Bars	Fruit, fruit purée, sugar, corn syrup, juice concentrate	90	18	1	1	1½ fruit
Dole Fruit and Yogurt Bars	Fruit, sugar, corn syrup	70	17	<1	1	1 fruit
Jell-O Pudding Pops	Sugar, corn syrup, dextrose	80	11	2	2	1 starch/bread
Jell-O Gelatin Pops	Sugar, corn syrup	35	8	0	1	½ fruit
Jell-O Fruit and Cream Bars	Sugar, fruit, dextrose, corn syrup	60	11	2	1	1 starch/bread

Table 14 Sample Nutrition Label

Chicken (Breast) Marsala with Vegetables

Nutrition Information (Single-serving pouch)	Per Serving
Serving size	9 oz
Servings per container	1
Calories	190
Protein	25 g
Carbohydrate	11 g
Fat	5 g
Sodium	850 mg
Potassium	220 mg

Percentage of U.S. Recommended Daily Allowances (U.S. RDA)

Protein	40	Thiamine	11
Vitamin A	22	Niacin	45
Vitamin C	16	Calcium	3
Riboflavin	11	Iron	5

Food exchanges (based on Exchange Lists for meal planning, American Diabetes Association, American Dietetic Association)
2½ lean meat
1 vegetable
½ starch/bread

The nutrition label can also tell you more specifically how a food product will fit into your meal plan. This labeling is optional for most foods unless the manufacturer makes a special nutritive claim about the product. If extra nutrients have been added, as in fortified products, then the package must provide composition information as well.

For those foods requiring labeling, government regulations specify that they list the following:

1. serving size given in commonly accepted measurements, such as ounces, cups, or teaspoons
2. number of servings per container
3. calories per serving and the weight (in grams) of protein, fat, carbohydrate, per serving

4. percentage of United States Recommended Daily Allowance (U.S. RDA) of vitamins A and C and certain other nutrients contained in that serving of food
5. identification of the type of fat a product contains, if the package makes a statement or claim about fats, such as "low in cholesterol or saturated fat"

A listing of sodium or potassium content is optional but is very often included.

Table 14 shows the typical format used for a nutrition label, and Table 15 defines some of the common food labeling terminology used on packages.

The nutrition label helps those with diabetes estimate how many exchanges are in that serving of food based on the calories, protein, fat, and carbohydrate per portion. The first step in converting nutritional labeling to exchanges is to determine if the serving size designated by the manufacturer is realistic for you. Because all nutrition information is based on a single serving size, you will need to make appropriate adjustments if one serving is either more or less than what is allowed in your meal plan. By comparing the label information with the calories, protein, fat, and carbohydrate in the exchange lists, you can determine the appropriate exchanges for one serving of what you plan to eat. For example, one 9-ounce package of the Chicken Marsala with Vegetables listed in Table 14 contains 190 calories, 11 grams of carbohydrate, 25 grams of protein, and 5 grams of fat. In terms of exchanges, this would translate into ½ starch/bread, 1 vegetable, and 2½ lean meat.

You need to know how to read labels in order to choose the right foods for optimal health. Make sure that you are not getting too many calories or too much sugar, fat, cholesterol, or sodium in your prepackaged and convenience foods.

Table 15   Understanding Food Labels

Term	Meaning
Light, lite	There are no precise definitions. If intended to be used for weight loss, must meet requirements for low- or reduced-calorie food
Low-calorie	No more than 40 calories per serving
Reduced-calorie	At least ⅓ fewer calories and nutritionally the same as the original product
Sugarless, sugar-free, no sugar	Product contains no sugars or nutritive carbohydrate sweeteners. For example, a milk product that contains lactose may be called "unsweetened" or "no sugar added" but not "sugar-free."
Unsweetened	Sweetened naturally, no sugars added
Artificially sweetened	Same restrictions as reduced-calorie or low-calorie foods
Diet, dietetic	Same as low-calorie or reduced-calorie; usually makes claim of special dietary usefulness, i.e., low-sodium or low-cholesterol
Imitation	Substitutes for another food but contains less than 2% of any of the nutrients required to be listed on the label
No added salt	No salt added during product preparation
Low-sodium	Less than 140 mg of sodium per serving
Very low sodium	Less than 35 mg of sodium per serving
Sodium-free	Less than 5 mg of sodium per serving
Fortified	Manufacturer adds nutrients not originally present in the food. For example, milk is fortified with vitamin D, margarine with vitamin A.

6

EXERCISE AND DIABETES

EXERCISE GOALS AND BENEFITS

We strongly advocate exercise as part of a successful diabetes management program. An ideal diabetes management plan achieves a balance among three factors: diet, exercise or activity, and medication. We now know that a person's ability to exercise and to derive benefit from exercise is very individual. Factors such as type of diabetes (insulin-dependent or non-insulin-dependent), current level of fitness, overall metabolic control, current nutritional status, age, and presence or absence of diabetic complications all have a significant impact on an individual's ability to exercise safely and effectively.

There are five main goals of an exercise program for all individuals with diabetes:

1. to maintain or improve cardiovascular (heart and blood vessel) fitness in order to reduce the risk factors for coronary heart disease
2. to assist in the control of blood glucose levels
3. to help lose weight or maintain an ideal weight
4. to allow safe and enjoyable participation in sports and physical activities
5. to reduce stress and anxiety
6. to improve self-image

Of great importance is the potential for exercise to decrease risk factors for coronary heart disease. Exercise may help protect against heart disease by favorably altering the level of high-density lipoprotein (HDL) cholesterol — the so-called good cholesterol (see glossary, p. 354). Aerobic exercise (such as brisk walking, swimming, and bicycling) three to four times per week has been shown to reduce the incidence of heart disease in the nondiabetic individual. Such exercise is even more important for persons with diabetes because of their added risk of heart disease.

For people with diabetes, regularly performed aerobic exercise improves the ability of muscle to respond to insulin and thus causes the muscles to take up more sugar. For people with insulin-dependent diabetes, improved insulin action may or may not lead to improved blood glucose control over time. However, blood glucose levels are generally reduced during and after an exercise session. As a result, there is the potential for decreased insulin requirements due to increased sensitivity of the active muscle to insulin. For people with non-insulin-dependent diabetes, some evidence suggests that regular aerobic exercise might improve blood sugar control by increasing the sensitivity of body cells to insulin, thus enhancing the effectiveness of an individual's insulin. Exercise may also decrease the amount of glucose released by the liver, helping to keep blood sugar levels normal.

A regular exercise program is an integral part of any weight loss program — especially when loss of body fat is desired and an increase in lean body mass is needed, as in the individual with non-insulin-dependent diabetes. In combination with cutting back on calories, exercise can lead to significant weight loss. People who have lost weight tend to regain fewer pounds if they continue to exercise regularly. In addition, people who exercise regularly tend to maintain lower body weights than those who do not.

A carefully planned exercise program will allow people with diabetes to experience the same benefits and enjoyment that people without diabetes gain from regular exercise. Improved self-image, appearance, and decreased psychological stress often accompany an exercise program.

EXERCISE AND INSULIN-DEPENDENT DIABETES

Because exercise adds to the blood-glucose-lowering effects of injected insulin, it enables a reduction in insulin dosages, providing at least short-term improvement in one's ability to handle glucose. This is a result of increased use of glucose and sensitivity to insulin. With the help of your physician, food intake and insulin dosage must be matched carefully to length and intensity of exercise to safely derive the most benefit in overall management of insulin-dependent diabetes.

You should check with your physician before embarking upon an exercise program. If you are over age thirty and have had diabetes for more than ten years, your first step should always be to obtain an exercise prescription from your physician. You should consider undergoing an exercise stress test to determine whether your heart is at risk during exercise. This test will also help you identify the heart rate you should work toward during exercise. The development of a prudent exercise program for the person with known coronary heart disease *must* be done under the guidance of an experienced exercise physiologist. Your level of glucose control also should be evaluated by your physician before you begin an exercise program. Exercise in the presence of poor metabolic control (insulin deficiency) can cause blood glucoses to rise further. The exercise physiologist who is a member of your health care team, or your physician, can recommend a conditioning program that fits your needs and capabilities. In planning the program, you need to discuss the following questions:

1. What kind of exercise will best help you accomplish your goals?
2. What kind of exercise will fit in with your lifestyle?
3. How often and how long should you exercise?
4. How hard or how intense should the exercise be?

The recommended intensity of your exercise program should be based on the exercise stress test and a target heart rate that your exercise physiologist or physician can prescribe. The stress test determines how much exercise you can do safely and how your heart and blood pressure respond to increased activity.

Blood glucose levels vary somewhat throughout the day, so it is ideal if you can exercise at approximately the same time each day. A consistent pattern is important — the same insulin dose, the same dietary pattern, and the same exercise pattern daily. It is advisable to exercise after a meal, keeping in mind the peak action of insulin. In general, you should not exercise when your insulin is exerting its maximum effect.

Blood glucose monitoring is an important tool for safe exercise. Monitoring your blood glucose before and after exercise is the best way to know how activity affects your blood glucose level. Records of pre- and post-exercise blood glucose levels and duration and intensity of the workout should be kept to establish patterns of how the particular exercise affects metabolic control. These patterns can be used by your health care professional to help you adapt food or insulin requirements to the time and amount of exercise that is planned for the first few months of a new program.

You may need to increase food intake before, during, or immediately after exercise. In general, most people with insulin-dependent diabetes tend to overeat on the day that they exercise to compensate for the exercise. This overeating may reduce the long-term benefits of improved metabolic control that can occur with exercise. The person taking insulin who exercises at about the same time daily should have a meal plan that provides enough calories to cover the exercise. If exercise is sporadic or less than daily, it is most appropriate to lower insulin doses and/or increase food intake to regulate blood glu-

Considerations

- Blood glucose monitoring is essential to document responses to exercise and to plan safe exercise sessions.
- It is important to have overall good blood glucose control before exercise.
- If blood glucose is more than 250 mg/dl and ketones are present, exercise will probably worsen control.
- If possible, exercise after meals or snacks to improve blood glucose response to food.
- Care must be taken not to eat too much food before exercise; however, if blood glucose is less than 100 mg/dl, eat a snack before exercising.
- Consider delaying eating extra food until after exercise.
- Base guidelines for increasing food intake on blood glucose levels before and after exercise and on how close to regularly scheduled meals and snacks exercise occurs.
- Exercise does not provide an opportunity to indulge in foods that are usually avoided, such as candy bars and desserts.
- Consider reducing insulin dosages before exercise.
- High blood glucose levels before exercise drop more with exercise than less elevated levels.
- Blood glucose can continue to drop for up to 30 hours after exercise, especially after vigorous or prolonged exercise or exercise that is done sporadically. This drop often occurs between 4 and 10 hours after exercise.
- Hypoglycemia during exercise or even 1 to 2 hours after exercise is relatively uncommon.
- Injection sites are not a major concern unless exercise is done immediately after injecting in an exercising limb.

cose levels. Table 16 provides general guidelines for food adjustments for various activities. However, you need to consult your physician, nurse, or exercise physiologist for the best recommendations for you.

Monitoring fluid intake is also *very* important during exercise. An adequate amount of fluid needs to be consumed before, during, and after exercise, particularly on warm days. For every pound of weight lost during exercise, you need 2 cups of fluid for replacement.

Exercise, especially long workouts, can increase the risk of hypoglycemia. Eating a small carbohydrate snack (based on the guidelines in Table 16) if blood sugar is lower than 90 mg/dl before exercising may be helpful. All individuals should carry adequate iden-

Table 16 How to Make Food Adjustments for Exercise (Insulin-Dependent Diabetes)*

Type of Exercise	Examples of Exercise	If Blood Glucose (in mg/dl) is	Increase Food Intake by	Suggested Foods to Use
Short duration of low to moderate intensity	Walking ½ mi or leisurely bicycling for <30 min	<80–99	10–15 g carbohydrate/h	1 fruit or 1 starch/bread exchange
		>100	Not necessary to increase food	
Moderate intensity	1 h of tennis, swimming, jogging, leisurely bicycling, gardening, golfing, or vacuuming	<80–100	25–50 g carbohydrate before exercise	½ meat sandwich with 1 milk and/or 1 fruit exchange
		100–180	10–15 g carbohydrate/h of exercise	1 fruit or 1 starch/bread exchange
		180–300†	Not necessary to increase food	
		>300†	Do not begin exercise until blood glucose levels are within target range.	

Type of Exercise	Examples of Exercise	If Blood Glucose (in mg/dl) is	Increase Food Intake by	Suggested Foods to Use
Strenuous activity or exercise	~1–2 h of football, hockey, racquetball, or basketball games; strenuous bicycling or swimming; shoveling heavy snow	<80–100	50 g carbohydrate; monitor blood glucose carefully	1 meat sandwich (2 slices bread) with 1 milk or fruit exchange
		100–180	25–50 g carbohydrate, depending on intensity and duration	½ meat sandwich with 1 milk and/or fruit exchange
		180–300†	10–15 g carbohydrate/h of exercise	1 fruit or 1 starch/bread exchange
		>300†	Do not begin exercise until blood glucose levels are within target range.	

*During period of exercise, individuals need to be sure to increase fluid intake. Self-monitoring of blood glucose is essential for all people to determine actual carbohydrate needs.

†Some individuals will experience hyperglycemia with pre-exercise values of ~250 mg/dl.

tification and a source of simple carbohydrate with them when they exercise in case a reaction occurs. Short-acting carbohydrates include juice, glucose tablets, and hard candies (see chapter 7). Another good idea is to exercise with a "buddy," someone who knows you have diabetes and knows how to help you if you have a reaction.

Hypoglycemia can also occur immediately following, or for up to 12 hours after, an exercise session. Be aware that blood glucose may continue to decrease after exercise, and be prepared. The body may need up to 24 hours to return to its pre-exercise state, particularly if the exercise is strenuous and not typical. Sometimes it is more important to eat a small snack after exercising than before.

EXERCISE AND NON-INSULIN-DEPENDENT DIABETES

Regular activity in conjunction with a weight-loss diet often controls non-insulin-dependent diabetes. In general, with increased activity there is an increase in sensitivity of body cells to insulin. Therefore, the cells are better able to store glucose and the body is more efficient in utilizing glucose. All of these things lead to better metabolic control.

Much of the advice for the individual with insulin-dependent diabetes is also appropriate for the non-insulin-dependent diabetic who is involved in an exercise program. It is helpful to measure blood sugar levels before and after exercise to adjust medication if necessary.

An extremely sedentary lifestyle, with only occasional bouts of exercise, does not improve diabetes control. Exercise and increased activity work best in controlling diabetes when they are part of your daily life. You can establish a routine of walking more, climbing stairs, doing housework, or working in your garden every day — all examples of lower-intensity exercise. A recent study at Stanford showed that people who used up 2000 calories per week through these lower-intensity activities reduced their death rate by 28 percent!

These lower-intensity forms of exercise allow your body to adjust safely to increased levels of activity over time. Your muscles, ligaments, and tendons become stronger and more flexible, gradually resulting in a musculoskeletal system that is less prone to injury. This is particularly important for the overweight diabetic, as excess pounds stress the weight-bearing joints — the hips, knees, and ankles — during exercise.

Diabetes control is best improved by regular aerobic activity.

Table 17   Caloric Cost of Various Activities

Activity	*Women* *130 pounds*	*Men* *180 pounds*
	(Calories per Minute)	
Aerobic	9.6	13.8
Bicycling		
6 mph	3.8	5.2
12 mph	10.0	13.8
Bowling	2.7	3.6
Calisthenics	3.9	5.4
Dancing		
slow	3.0	4.2
fast	10.0	13.7
Golf (walking and carrying bag)	5.0	7.0
Running or jogging		
5 mph	8.0	11.0
7.5 mph	11.3	15.8
Skating (ice or roller)	4.4	6.1
Skiing		
downhill	5.0	7.2
cross-country	7.0	9.7
Swimming (fast and freestyle)	7.6	10.4
Tennis		
singles	6.4	8.9
doubles	3.8	5.2
Walking		
3 mph	3.4	5.2
4 mph	5.5	7.7
up stairs	8.5	11.8
Weight training	6.1	8.4

Aerobic activity is continuous, rhythmic exercise that gives your whole body a workout. If your physician gives you the green light, choose an aerobic activity that will get your heart rate up and make you actually sweat. Choose one of the aerobic activities in Table 17 or any other aerobic activity that fits your lifestyle. Four to five exercise sessions per week will optimize fat loss, increase lean body mass, and burn the appropriate number of calories needed to lose weight.

EXERCISE INFORMATION FOR PERSONS WITH NON-INSULIN-DEPENDENT DIABETES

Benefits

Exercise
- Increases sensitivity of body cells to insulin.
- Enables cells to store glucose better.
- Lowers the amount of glucose produced by the liver, helping keep blood glucose values normal.
- Reduces body fat and increases muscle. Muscle cells use more glucose than fat cells.
- Can result in a change in the distribution of fat — a decrease in the waist-to-hip ratio. People with this type of fat distribution are less likely to have high insulin levels, elevated blood fats, and high blood pressure.
- Can be an adjunct to diet to assist with weight control.
- Can lower cholesterol and triglyceride levels.
- Can lower blood pressure.

Risks

- Injuries to feet can occur, especially if nerve damage is present.
- Coronary heart attacks can occur.
- Blood pressure during exercise may rise higher in persons with diabetes than in persons without diabetes.
- Problems with eyes, kidneys, and lungs may be worsened.

IMPORTANT TIPS

- Commit to a minimum number of exercise sessions per week and stick with it.
- Keep a record of your weight and measurements. Measure your chest, waist, hips, and thighs to watch them slim down as you become more fit.
- Measure your resting heart rate. The fact that it slows down is a definite sign that you are becoming more fit.
- Become aware of how many calories you are burning when you exercise. If you walk at a pace of about 3 miles per hour, you burn the number of calories equal to 0.03 times your body weight in pounds per minute. Thus, a 200-pound person would burn 6 calories per minute walking 3 miles per hour. If you walk more

Considerations

- Check with a physician before beginning an exercise program.
- Because benefits of exercise on glucose are transient, exercise has to be done on a regular and long-term basis.
- Exercise done in the evening can still have beneficial effects on blood glucose levels the next morning.
- Benefits of exercise are lost when no exercise is performed for a 3-day period.
- Do not compensate for the increased calories used during and after exercise by being less active than usual at other times of the day. This is often a problem if calories are severely restricted.
- Exercise can result in an increase in appetite and, therefore, calorie intake. Care must be taken not to increase food intake.
- To be beneficial, exercise must be performed at least three times a week.
- Persons with blood glucose values of less than 200 mg/dl have a greater glycemic benefit from exercise than persons with a higher blood glucose level.
- Persons taking sulfonylureas and who have normal blood glucose values may need to reduce or omit the sulfonylurea before exercising.

slowly, you will burn fewer calories per minute. Ideally, an exercise session would burn between 350 and 500 calories. Avoid the temptation of rewarding yourself with a snack — one fast-food burger is worth 500 to 600 calories!

- Try varying the type of exercise that you do to prevent boredom and burnout. You can, for example, alternate your walking routes. Find a partner or join a class. Having company can boost morale and motivation.
- If the weather does not permit outdoor exercise, try mall walking. There are now many organized clubs of mall walkers catering to different levels of capability.
- Aqua-aerobics (in swimming pools) can provide a good low-impact form of exercise.
- Try exercise or jazzercise programs on television, but be careful to choose the proper level of intensity. Music can make exercise more fun.
- Keep an exercise diary to provide you with the positive feedback of your accomplishments.
- Hang in there — you *can* do it!

7

MONITORING
AND CONTROL
OF BLOOD
GLUCOSES

IMPORTANCE OF NORMAL BLOOD GLUCOSES

One of the major goals for people with diabetes is to maintain blood glucose at the optimal level determined by themselves and their physician. This is important to prevent medical emergencies associated with high blood glucose levels (ketoacidosis) and low blood glucose levels (hypoglycemic episodes) and to increase overall health and well-being. Optimal glucose control is achieved by the proper balance of diet, exercise, and medication. This chapter provides an overview of glucose monitoring and management. Monitoring of your glucose levels will help you understand your body's response to dietary and exercise changes.

MONITORING GLUCOSE LEVELS

The key to stable metabolic control is the maintenance of a balance among diet, activity, and medication (insulin or oral hypoglycemic agent). Blood glucose levels fluctuate as you go about your daily routine. Eating causes the blood glucose level to go up; activity (exercise) causes it to fall. When insulin (or an oral hypoglycemic agent) is working properly in the body, it helps stabilize blood glucose levels. In order to control blood glucose levels, it is helpful to monitor them several times a day. This can be done by measuring the amount of glucose in the blood or urine.

Urine Testing Urine test results reflect what has happened to an individual's glucose levels during the preceding time period. The

78

kidneys filter excess glucose from the bloodstream, and it then passes into the urine when blood glucose levels have exceeded the kidney's threshold. Because it takes several hours for the kidney to remove extra glucose from the blood and send it into the urine, the actual blood glucose levels have likely changed by the time a urine sample is tested. Thus, urine results can be helpful in identifying trends in glucose control. If the test is positive, it tells you that your blood glucose was high several hours before. However, urine testing does not yield an absolute glucose value and, therefore, can be confusing at times — especially when interpreting hypoglycemic symptoms.

Blood Testing   Blood testing is a more precise way of monitoring changes in blood glucose levels, particularly at times when adjustments are actively being made in your treatment plan. With the advent of home blood-glucose monitoring equipment, the individual with diabetes is now able to monitor blood glucose levels regularly. To measure, you prick your finger and place a drop of blood on a test strip. The strip changes to one of several colors, depending on how much glucose is in the blood. This color is then matched to a standard reference chart or interpreted by a meter that reads the test strips more precisely, yielding a specific glucose value.

Using the proper technique, self-monitoring is the best method of determining the blood glucose level at any given time. If you want to determine the effect of a change in insulin or diet — say, increasing your insulin or eating a special meal out — measuring your blood glucose before and after the change can be useful. Or, if you are concerned about the possibility of an insulin reaction during sports or while driving, you can check your blood glucose before and/or during the activity and have a snack to treat or prevent a low blood glucose reaction. Rather than guessing or speculating about the effect of treatment change on your diabetes, you will be able to make appropriate modifications based on real measurements.

Regardless of the method of monitoring you use, keeping a diary, in which you write down time and amount of medication (insulin or oral agent), the results of glucose tests, activity level, and food intake, is invaluable. Examples of two different self-monitoring diaries appear on pp. 78 and 82–83. One provides space to record diet and exercise patterns, and the other provides space simply to record insulin dose and blood or urine test results. The information in the diary is important in helping you and your physician or diabetes specialist work out any changes that are needed in your treatment regimen.

Self-Monitoring Diary A

Date	Diet and Calorie Log Goal: ____ calories/day					Exercise	Glucose Monitoring		Rx	Notes
	Breakfast	Lunch	Dinner	Snacks	Total Calories	Type/ Duration	Blood/urine Time/result		Time	
Monday										
Calories										
Tuesday										
Calories										
Wednesday										
Calories										
Thursday										
Calories										
Friday										
Calories										
Saturday										
Calories										
Sunday										
Calories										

For self-monitoring of blood glucose levels to be truly effective, the results recorded in your diary need to be interpreted and integrated into your management plan with the help of your physician or nurse.

MEDICATION

Although Type I and Type II diabetes share the common symptom of high blood glucose or hypoglycemia, the methods of treatment differ. If you have Type I diabetes, you require daily injections of insulin to replace the hormone that is no longer produced by the body. Without insulin, life cannot be sustained. If you have Type II diabetes your body still produces insulin, but the insulin does not work as efficiently as it should. Thus, daily management may consist of a weight-loss program, oral hypoglycemic agents (diabetes pills), or insulin injections.

Insulin   Insulin is a hormone made by beta cells in the pancreas. Insulin carried in the blood enables the body's cells to utilize food properly — particularly carbohydrates. Insulin must be injected because it is a protein that would be broken down by the digestive system if taken by mouth. Insulin stays in the bloodstream for several hours after it is injected.

Insulin's effect on blood glucose levels is influenced by the type of insulin used (short-acting, intermediate-acting, or long-acting), the number of units taken, the time of day when it is taken, and the site of the injection. The insulin, dietary intake, and activity level interact to produce a blood glucose level at a given time. It is important to know three things about the insulin you take:

- when it begins to work after an injection
- the onset and length of time that it will work most efficiently
- when the effect begins to lessen or go away (duration)

Figure 3 shows the different types of insulin and their different time schedules. Your physician or nurse will decide which type of insulin regimen best fits your lifestyle and individual needs. Your optimal daily schedule may require one to several injections per day. You may be mixing a short-acting with an intermediate- or long-acting insulin for optimal metabolic control. When taken at the same time, the mixed insulins work together to control blood glucose immediately after injection, as well as over a longer period of time.

Oral Hypoglycemics   Those with Type II, or non-insulin-dependent, diabetes often make more than adequate amounts of insulin. However, the insulin may not work efficiently enough to control blood glucose levels. The oral hypoglycemic agents enable the body

Self-Monitoring Diary B

Date	Insulin Type	Breakfast		Lunch		Dinner		Bedtime		Ketone Tests	Notes
		Insulin Dose	Blood and/or Urine Glucose Testing	Insulin Dose	Blood and/or Urine Glucose Testing	Insulin Dose	Blood and/or Urine Glucose Testing	Insulin Dose	Blood and/or Urine Glucose Testing	Results / Time	
	R / N / L										
	R / N / L										
	R / N / L										

For self-monitoring of blood glucose levels to be truly effective, the results recorded in your diary need to be interpreted and integrated into your management plan with your physician or nurse.

R = regular or short-acting insulin

N/L = "NPH" or "Lente," intermediate-acting insulin

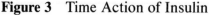

Figure 3 Time Action of Insulin

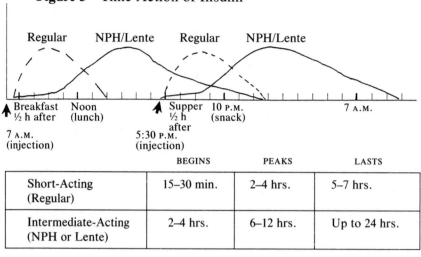

	BEGINS	PEAKS	LASTS
Short-Acting (Regular)	15–30 min.	2–4 hrs.	5–7 hrs.
Intermediate-Acting (NPH or Lente)	2–4 hrs.	6–12 hrs.	Up to 24 hrs.

to use the insulin that is available more efficiently. Oral hypoglycemic agents act by increasing insulin secretion and enhancing insulin's effectiveness. Along with proper dietary control (the right kind of foods and weight loss if necessary), oral hypoglycemics can be very effective in lowering blood glucose levels in some people with non-insulin-dependent diabetes. The more commonly used oral hypoglycemic agents include glyburide and glipizide compounds.

HIGH BLOOD GLUCOSE: HYPERGLYCEMIA

High blood glucose is a condition known as hyperglycemia. If your blood glucose levels rise to 250 mg/dl or greater, you may experience some symptoms of hyperglycemia: increased urination, increased thirst, tiredness, blurred vision, weight loss without dieting, infections, and numbness or burning of the hands and feet.

Hyperglycemia can occur when there is an imbalance among insulin, food, and activity. If you suspect that your glucose level is high, test your blood or urine glucose. If it is above the level your physician has identified as optimal for you, try to determine the cause: Did you receive the right amount of medication during the day? Did you recently eat a larger meal than usual, or one with more simple sugars? Has your activity level changed dramatically? Are you in a stressful situation or ill? It is important to determine why your blood glucoses are elevated and to contact your physician if they remain high for a prolonged period. Certain medications may also elevate blood glucose levels, so be sure to discuss their use with your physician.

Ketoacidosis If insulin deficiency is severe enough, blood glucose levels will continue to rise. When blood glucose levels are in excess of 300 mg/dl, little or no glucose can be used as a source of energy. As a result, increased fat breakdown occurs and the body must rely on the breakdown of stored fat for energy. When this happens, compounds known as ketones are sent into the blood. It is important to test your urine for ketones during this time to avoid a buildup in the body and produce a condition called diabetic ketoacidosis. Symptoms of ketoacidosis include nausea, vomiting, stomach cramps, deep and rapid breathing, and a fruity odor to the breath. Anything more than a trace of ketones in the urine may be a warning sign of potential diabetic ketoacidosis. Call your physician to find out what to do to bring your blood glucoses back down to an optimal level. Individuals with Type II diabetes rarely become insulin-deficient to the extent that ketoacidosis develops.

LOW BLOOD SUGAR: HYPOGLYCEMIA

Hypoglycemia results from abnormally low blood glucose and is also known as an insulin reaction. Hypoglycemic symptoms often occur when the blood sugar is below 60 mg/dl, or if there is a rapid drop in blood glucose levels. Hypoglycemia can occur very rapidly and progress if left untreated. The most common cause of hypoglycemia is too little food in the body when compared to the amount of medication that has been taken. It occurs, for example, when a person with insulin-dependent diabetes takes insulin and then eats a meal later than usual, skips a meal, or eats too little at meal time. Hypoglycemia rarely occurs in the person with non-insulin-dependent diabetes taking oral hypoglycemic agents. Increased activity will also sometimes cause hypoglycemia because exercise burns some of the glucose in the blood. Hypoglycemia can occur during or after exercise, particularly prolonged workouts.

Alcohol, too, can cause hypoglycemia by interfering with the body's natural ability to raise blood glucose if it is low. Alcohol can be especially troublesome if taken on an empty stomach; it should be

Table 18 The Quick Guide to Blood Glucose Levels

HYPOGLYCEMIA (can come on suddenly)				HYPERGLYCEMIA (usually develops slowly)
Very Low (under 40) Severe insulin reaction	Low (40–65) Mild insulin reaction	Normal (65–140)	High (250–350)	Very High (over 350)
SYMPTOMS	SYMPTOMS		SYMPTOMS	SYMPTOMS
■ Confusion	■ Shakiness and nervousness		■ Extreme thirst	Same as for high blood sugar and possibly:
■ Personality changes	■ Rapid pulse		■ Frequent urination	■ Nausea
■ Staggering	■ Perspiration, cold and clammy skin		■ Fatigue	■ Stomach cramps
■ Slurred speech	■ Feeling of weakness or faintness		■ Vision changes	■ Dry mouth, dehydration
■ Convulsions	■ Blurred or double vision		■ Dry skin and mouth	■ Fruity breath
■ Loss of consciousness	■ Tingling of hands, lips, or tongue			■ Ketones in urine
	■ Headache			■ Weight loss
	■ Sudden hunger			■ Deep and rapid breathing
				■ Drowsiness
				■ Unconsciousness

HYPOGLYCEMIA (can come on suddenly)		Normal	HYPERGLYCEMIA (usually develops slowly)	
Very Low (under 40) Severe insulin reaction	*Low (40–65)* Mild insulin reaction	*(65–140)*	*High (250–350)*	*Very High (over 350)*
CAUSES • Ignored or inadequately treated mild hypoglycemia	CAUSES • Too little food (late, insufficient, or missed meals) • Too much insulin or diabetes pills • Too much exercise without food • Alcohol (especially on an empty stomach)		CAUSES • Too much food • Wrong kinds of food • Illness, infection, or injury • Emotional stress • Too little diabetes medication • Previously undiagnosed diabetes	CAUSES • Same as for high blood sugar
TREATMENT *If person is awake,* treat as you would a mild insulin reaction. *If person is unconscious:* • Dial 911 or fire department paramedics. • Rub Monogel, Instaglucose, or Cake-Mate between cheek and gum or . . . • Inject glucagon.	TREATMENT Simple sugars such as: • Orange or apple juice or regular soft drink (4 oz) • 5–7 jelly beans, gum drops, or sugar cubes • 2–3 glucose tablets. Repeat if needed. If more than 30 minutes until meal, eat a snack (cheese and crackers or half a sandwich).		TREATMENT • Follow meal plan. • Take medication properly. • Notify doctor to treat underlying illness or infection or adjust amount of medication.	TREATMENT • Test urine for ketones. • Notify your doctor, who can tell you how to treat yourself or where to find treatment quickly.

consumed infrequently and in conjunction with a meal or snack. Be sure to check with your physician to determine whether an occasional alcoholic drink in your meal plan is safe for you. Chapter 4 provides general guidelines (based on information from the American Diabetes Association) on how to count alcoholic beverages in your meal plan.

Signs and symptoms of hypoglycemia can include dizziness, nausea, increased perspiration, headaches, irritability, drowsiness, blurred vision, hunger, shakiness, decreased coordination, and confusion. Loss of consciousness and seizures can occur if the early signs and symptoms are disregarded. If you think that your blood glucose might be low, do a blood test to determine if you are right. If you are unable to test your blood, assume you are experiencing hypoglycemia and treat the symptoms.

Treat mild to moderate hypoglycemia (blood glucose of 65 mg/dl or less) by eating 15 grams of simple carbohydrate. Best choices include:

   4 ounces of orange juice

   4 ounces of apple juice

   2 ounces of grape juice

If juices are not available, try one of the following:

   3 glucose tablets (quick-acting and easy to transport)

   4 ounces of nondiet cola

   2 tablespoons of raisins

   1 tablespoon of honey

   5 to 7 pieces of small hard candy such as Life Savers, jelly beans, or gum drops

After taking in some type of simple sugar, recheck your blood 10 to 15 minutes later. Your symptoms should be disappearing as your blood glucose rises. If not, or if your blood glucose is still less than 60 mg/dl, treat yourself again with the same amount of food, tablets, or beverage and wait another 10 to 15 minutes. If your low blood glucose and/or symptoms persist, contact your physician.

Respond to low blood glucose episodes even if your meal time is near, so that your symptoms do not progress or become worse. Moving your meal time ahead, or eating the fruit portion of your meal a few minutes early, is ideal. If these measures do not work well, consult your physician for advice.

If early hypoglycemia is not treated, it can progress to more severe hypoglycemia, in which blood sugar drops below 40 mg/dl. Symptoms at this lower level may include confusion, lack of coordination, slurred speech, and behavior changes. Unconsciousness can result from these lower levels because sufficient glucose is not available to allow for normal brain function. Check with your physician regarding the recommended emergency procedures for treating a severe insulin reaction, as well as for methods to prevent such episodes.

The following precautions and reminders will help prevent hypoglycemia and its complications:

1. Eat your meals completely and on time.
2. Wear some kind of bracelet or carry other forms of identification that will help determine the type of diabetes you have and the type of medication you are taking.
3. Carry some form of fast-acting carbohydrate with you, especially when exercising.
4. Drink alcoholic beverages only in moderation and with meals.
5. Pay attention to your "peak" times, when insulin is acting at its strongest.
6. Carry a snack for exercise workouts and periods of increased activity.
7. Plan ahead and be prepared so that you are not caught short when your blood glucose becomes low.

Table 18 offers you, at a glance, the symptoms, causes, and treatments for both hyperglycemia and hypoglycemia.

PART TWO

THE RECIPES

HOW TO USE THESE RECIPES

THE PURPOSE of this cookbook is to provide a wide variety of new and exciting recipes that show you how to eat lightly and wisely every day — as well as how to entertain and splurge occasionally in a healthful way. The recipes come from many sources with decidedly ethnic and regional flavors. Our gourmet approach emphasizes fresh herbs and seasonings and subtle flavors that do not overwhelm the palate the way too much salt, sugar, and fat can.

We have given a great deal of attention to the nutritional composition of these recipes, developing each of them with these guidelines in mind:

• *Reduced total fat.* Minimal use of oils and margarines has held the total fat content of many main dishes, salads, desserts, and side dishes to under 30 percent of total calories. Most side dishes and salads contain 5 grams of fat or less per serving; desserts contain 5 to 7 grams of fat or less per serving. Most main dishes contain 15 grams of fat or less per serving. The recipes that are slightly higher in fat include suggestions for low-fat foods to accompany the meal so that the total fat content of the meal does not exceed 30 percent.

• *Reduced cholesterol and saturated fat.* The cholesterol content of our recipes does not exceed 150 milligrams per serving, with the exception of two recipes that contain shrimp which are slightly higher. Wherever possible we have substituted egg whites for whole eggs or minimized the use of eggs. Foods from animal and vegetable sources that are high in saturated fat, such as butter, cream, and coconut, are not included.

• *Increased fiber and complex carbohydrates.* Recipes for more meatless main meals, and the use of whole grains, beans, and pastas give you ideas for increasing your fiber intake.

• *Reduced salt and the use of high-sodium ingredients.* Most of our recipes contain 400 milligrams of sodium or less per serving. We have indicated with an asterisk those recipes containing more sodium, allowing the cook to plan the rest of the meal, or even the rest of the day, to be lower in sodium.

• *Limited use of calorie-containing and alternative sweeteners.* The use of sugar, honey, or molasses does not exceed ¾ teaspoon per serving. And we have been careful not to overload recipes with too much fruit juice or fresh or dried fruit, so that simple sugar content is not excessive. Fructose is used in some of our recipes in amounts specified by the American Diabetes Association (see chapter 2). We use noncaloric sweeteners in a few recipes to provide a sweeter flavor without added calories and simple sugar.

The nutrient analysis that accompanies the recipes will help you fit them into your own meal plan. We've also provided exchanges for individual servings, based on the Exchange Lists for Meal Planning from the American Diabetes Association/American Dietetic Association. Calculating exchanges for recipes is somewhat subjective, but what is calculated should most accurately reflect the ingredients of a recipe as well as its calorie and nutrient content. We have tried to assign exchanges to our recipes according to their ingredients and nutrient content, but be aware that there may be other options. This is particularly true when you have mixed dishes with many ingredients. We have tried to use only full exchanges and used half exchanges only when necessary.

We have also included a large number of easy, quick, and microwave recipes to meet the needs of busy cooks. Easy recipes are those that take less than 20 minutes to prepare. Quick recipes are those that take less than 30 minutes to prepare and cook. You'll find the labels EASY, QUICK, and MICROWAVE to the right of the recipe titles.

All of our recipes have been developed, tested, tasted, and modified in the research kitchen of the Clinical Research Center at the University of California. And many of our friends and family have "road tested" them over the last four years. There may be times when your yield varies from that given in the recipe. Accuracy in measurements, particular measuring utensils, cutting preference (slicing, dicing, chopping), moisture loss, and oven temperature can account for these differences. So, as we do even in our research kitchen, allow for some minor variations, and *bon appétit!*

HOW TO STOCK YOUR CUPBOARD

Staples

Baking powder
Baking soda
Barley
Broth, beef and chicken, canned or bouillon cubes, preferably
    low-sodium
Bulgur
Cereals, hot and cold high-fiber (7-grain, oatmeal, oat bran,
    wheat, and wheat bran products)
Cornstarch
Crackers, whole wheat or graham
Dried fruits, such as raisins and dates
Flour, unbleached all-purpose and whole wheat
Fructose
Gelatin, unflavored
Herbs and spices (see pp. 30–31)
Honey
Milk, canned, evaporated, skimmed
Milk, nonfat dry
Oil, vegetable, nonstick cooking spray
Oil, vegetable, poly- and monounsaturated (see Table 5)
Pasta, whole wheat and vegetable
Peanut butter, natural style, no added fats or sugar
Popcorn
Rice, brown and white
Salmon, canned in water
Soy sauce, preferably low-sodium
Sugar substitute
Tomatoes, canned
Tomato (marinara) sauce, low-fat
Tomato paste

Tuna, canned in water

Vinegars, distilled white, red wine, herb- and fruit-flavored, balsamic

HOW TO STOCK YOUR REFRIGERATOR

Staples

Bread, 100 percent whole grain
Cheese, low-fat or part-skim
Chicken broth, preferably low-sodium homemade
Eggs (whites)/egg substitute
Fruit spread or pure fruit jam
Fresh fruits and vegetables in season
Margarine, brands low in saturated fats (see Table 5)
Mayonnaise, reduced-calorie
Milk, low-fat or nonfat
Mustard
Salad dressings, light or low-calorie
Tortillas, corn
Tortillas, flour, made with vegetable oil, low in saturated fat
Yogurt, nonfat

And Any of the Following

Chicken or turkey breasts
Fish, shellfish
Frozen desserts, low-fat, low-calorie, or sugar-free
Ground sirloin or lean ground beef
Ground turkey
Turkey sausage

MICROWAVE TIPS

Microwave cooking is quick and easy if you know the basics. It is also a great way to preserve the flavor and nutrients in foods. Microwave ovens are extremely versatile and offer an ideal way to cook many foods such as fish, chicken, and vegetables — and, of course, they are most convenient for reheating and defrosting.

Here are some tips for using a microwave:

1. Cooking vegetables — It is important to cut vegetables to a uniform size and thickness to provide even cooking. Thicker vegetables, especially potatoes, should be pierced with a knife to prevent skins from exploding.

   Careful arrangement of unevenly shaped food, such as potatoes, in the microwave is important to assure proper cooking. Place thinner, less dense areas toward the center of the microwave and thicker, denser areas to the outside, where microwave cooking begins first. The denser parts, which take longer to cook, will receive more microwave energy and be done at about the same time as the less dense parts of food.

   For maximum nutrient and flavor retention, cook vegetables in a small amount of water in a microwave-safe dish, covered tightly with plastic wrap. Pierce the plastic before removing to prevent steam burns. Because steam actually cooks the vegetables, it is important to allow standing time to complete the cooking process. Cooking and standing times will vary with the type of vegetable and the type of microwave oven. Check your owner's manual or a microwave cookbook for precise times.

2. Cooking meat, fish, and poultry — Like vegetables, it is best to cut meat portions into uniform size and thickness. Small pieces will cook more consistently and uniformly than large ones. Higher protein foods, such as meat, fish, and poultry, are generally better if cooked on a lower power to prevent toughness. You can cook tender cuts of meat, however, on high. Cook less tender cuts of meat in some liquid, on medium heat, for a longer period. Allow for some standing time to finish cooking, and check your owner's manual to determine exact cooking times.

In general, the following cooking times should apply:
Beef: 10 to 12 minutes per pound of roast
      2 to 4 minutes per pound of ground meat patty
Chicken/turkey: 6 to 7 minutes per pound
Fish: 3 to 5 minutes per pound

HOW TO ADAPT YOUR OWN RECIPE

1. To reduce cholesterol content of recipes:
- Use vegetable oils instead of animal fats, such as lard and butter.
- Use margarine instead of butter.
- Substitute 2 egg whites for one whole egg, or use a commercial egg substitute.
- Use more vegetables, legumes, and grains and less meat in a recipe (e.g., chili with more beans or soup with more split peas but less ham).
- Use a soy-based product to replace part or all of the meat in a recipe (such as Tofu-Tempeh Lasagna or Shrimp and Feta with Tofu).
- Use nonfat milk products instead of whole milk products.

2. To reduce the fat content of recipes:
- Use reduced-calorie mayonnaise and salad dressings.
- Blend cottage cheese or yogurt with nonfat milk to make a sour cream type of topping.
- Replace regular whipping cream with low-calorie whipping cream or a small amount of vanilla low-fat yogurt.
- Remove all visible fat from meat and skin from poultry before cooking.
- Decrease oil in marinades and salad dressings and increase vinegars, water, and seasonings.
- Use foods (fish, artichokes, beans, etc.) canned in their own juice or with water; avoid foods canned in heavy oil.
- De-fat meat drippings by refrigerating or freezing them and skimming the fat off the top.
- Decrease the amount of fat used in baked goods by one third to one half and increase the fluids called for in the recipe to reach the desired consistency.
- Cheese that is finely grated or thinly sliced goes further.
- Pour some of the fat off the top of the "natural" peanut butters before using.

3. To reduce the sodium content of recipes:
- Use low-salt or no-salt-added products.
- Increase your use of herbs and spices in place of salt in recipes. (See Herb and Spice Combinations on pp. 30–31 and Savory Seasonings on p. 291.)

- Use fresh foods whenever possible in place of canned or processed foods (soup mixes, cured meats, etc.) or rinse canned foods (tuna, vegetables) with water.
- Do not add salt to water when cooking pasta or other foods.

4. To reduce the sugar content of recipes:
- Decrease the amount of sugar called for in traditional recipes by *at least* one third; substitute fruit juices, nectars, or puréed fruits.
- Use fruit canned in water or canned in its own juice.
- Use noncaloric sweeteners if needed to increase the sweetness of a recipe without added calories. (We have found that most baked desserts and sweet breads require at least ¾ teaspoon of sugar per serving to achieve a desirable flavor.)

8

SIPS, DIPS, CHIPS, AND APPETIZERS

SERVE THESE RECIPES prior to the first course to stimulate appetite. Thanks to recent cooking trends, mundane high-salt, high-fat fare such as onion dip, potato chips, and cheese spreads are a thing of the past. Our recipes for Tempeh Pâté, Garlic Lover's Dip, and Spicy Salsa reflect changing American tastes. Try our No-Fry Tortilla Chips, Toasted Pita Chips, fresh vegetable recipes, or a sliced, fresh, whole wheat baguette as a low-fat accompaniment.

Banana Smoothies
Berry Spritzer
Spiced Cocoa

Bean Dip
Chili con Queso
Cottage Cheese Caraway
　Spread
Eggplant Relish Italiano
Garlic Lover's Dip
Guacamole
Pesto Dip

Salmon Spread
Spicy Salsa
Tempeh Pâté

No-Fry Tortilla Chips
Pasta Chips
Toasted Pita Chips

Crab Mornay
Spicy Seafood Wontons
Spinach Appetizers

BANANA SMOOTHIES ———————————————— QUICK

Blender drinks are easy to make and healthful. Prepare them the night before and reblend before serving in the morning for a quick breakfast. Substitute fresh fruit in season.

Combine all ingredients in a blender or food processor until smooth.

Version 1
- ½ cup low-fat milk
- ¼ cup low-fat vanilla yogurt
- ½ banana
- ¼ teaspoon vanilla
- **Dash of cinnamon**

Yield: 1 serving, 1 cup
One Serving = 1 cup

Calories: 178
Protein: 7 g
Fat: 3 g
Carbohydrate: 32 g
Fiber: 1.3 g
Cholesterol: 12 mg
Sodium: 97 mg
Potassium: 535 mg

Exchange: 1 fruit
1 low-fat milk

Version 2
- ½ cup low-fat milk
- ¼ cup low-fat vanilla yogurt
- ½ banana
- ½ cup orange juice
  (preferably freshly squeezed)

Yield: 1 serving, 1½ cups
One Serving = 1½ cups

Calories: 233
Protein: 8 g
Fat: 3 g
Carbohydrate: 45 g
Fiber: 1.6 g
Cholesterol: 12 mg
Sodium: 99 mg
Potassium: 770 mg

Exchange: 2 fruit
1 low-fat milk

Version 3
- ½ cup low-fat milk
- ¼ cup low-fat vanilla yogurt
- ½ banana
- ¼ cup strawberries, sliced fresh or frozen, unsweetened

Yield: 1 serving, 1 cup
One Serving = 1 cup

Calories: 188
Protein: 8 g
Fat: 3 g
Carbohydrate: 34 g

Fiber: 2 g
Cholesterol: 12 mg
Sodium: 98 mg
Potassium: 601 mg

Exchange: 1 fruit
1 low-fat milk

BERRY SPRITZER _____ QUICK

Two reasons to try this spritzer other than its great taste: it contains considerably less sugar than commercial versions, and the fresh strawberries contain fiber.

> **1 cup strawberries, hulled**
> **½ cup unsweetened apple juice**
> **½ cup club soda or sparkling water**
> **Mint leaves for garnish**

1. Blend strawberries and apple juice in a blender or food processor until smooth.
2. Add club soda and blend thoroughly.
3. Pour into 2 glasses. Garnish with mint leaves.

Yield: 2 servings, 1½ cups
One Serving = ¾ cup

Calories: 52	Fiber: 1.7 g
Protein: <1 g	Cholesterol: 0
Fat: <1 g	Sodium: 15 mg
Carbohydrate: 12 g	Potassium: 199 mg

Exchange: 1 fruit

SPICED COCOA _____ QUICK

This hot cocoa is high in calcium but low in fat and sugar because we have replaced the whole milk and cream with nonfat milk and the sugar with a noncaloric sweetener.

> **2½ teaspoons unsweetened cocoa powder**
> **Drop of vanilla**
> **6 ounces nonfat milk, heated**
> **2 packages Equal**
> **1 tablespoon Whipped Topping (optional, p. 297)**
> **Nutmeg for garnish (optional)**

1. Combine cocoa and vanilla in a mug. Add the warm milk and mix thoroughly.
2. Stir in Equal.
3. Add Whipped Topping and nutmeg, if desired. Serve immediately.

Yield: 1 serving, 6 ounces
One Serving = 6 ounces, plain

Calories: 90
Protein: 7 g
Fat: 1 g
Carbohydrate: 13 g

Fiber: 0
Cholesterol: 3 mg
Sodium: 95 mg
Potassium: 379 mg

Exchange: 1 nonfat milk

BEAN DIP _____ QUICK

This dip makes a marvelous burrito filling. Simply spoon the bean dip inside a warm tortilla and roll up. For an even easier bean dip, combine several tablespoons of salsa with refried beans and serve with tortilla chips.

¼ cup diced green chilies
¼ cup tomato sauce or mild chili salsa (green or red)
4 green onions, chopped
¼–½ teaspoon cumin
½ clove garlic, minced
1 can (30 ounces) refried beans
Freshly grated low-fat cheese (optional)

1. Combine chilies, tomato sauce, onions, and seasonings in a saucepan and cook until onions are tender.
2. Add beans and cook approximately 8 minutes.
3. Serve either hot or cold; top with grated low-fat cheese if desired.

Yield: 16 servings, 4 cups
One Serving = 4 tablespoons (without cheese)

Calories: 76
Protein: 4 g
Fat: 1 g
Carbohydrate: 12 g

Fiber: 6.4 g*
Cholesterol: 0
Sodium: 302 mg
Potassium: 262 mg

Exchange: 1 starch/bread

*Good source of dietary fiber

CHILI CON QUESO ────────────────────────── QUICK

Serve this dip with a bowl of No-Fry Tortilla Chips (p. 111).

3 green onions, chopped
1 clove garlic, pressed or minced
3 tablespoons water
1 can (4 ounces) chopped green chilies, drained
1 can (8 ounces) stewed tomatoes, drained
⅛ teaspoon cayenne pepper
1 cup freshly grated low-fat Monterey Jack cheese

1. Sauté onions and garlic in water until soft.
2. Add chilies, tomatoes, and cayenne pepper. Cook on low heat for 8 to 10 minutes, stirring often.
3. Stir in cheese until melted.

Yield: 8 servings, 2 cups
One Serving = ¼ cup

Calories: 64	Fiber: 0.6 g
Protein: 4 g	Cholesterol: 8 mg
Fat: 4 g	Sodium: 350 mg
Carbohydrate: 4 g	Potassium: 124 mg

Exchange: 1 vegetable
          1 fat

COTTAGE CHEESE CARAWAY SPREAD ─────────── EASY

A great accompaniment to Toasted Pita Chips (p. 112).

2 cups freshly grated low-fat   **⅓ cup chopped green onion**
    Monterey Jack cheese   **1 teaspoon caraway seeds**
1 cup low-fat cottage cheese   **¼ teaspoon salt**
½ cup dry white wine

1. Combine all ingredients in a blender or food processor until smooth.
2. Chill before serving.

Yield: 14 servings, 3½ cups
One Serving = ¼ cup

Calories: 80
Protein: 6 g
Fat: 5 g
Carbohydrate: 1 g

Fiber: 0.1 g
Cholesterol: 17 mg
Sodium: 206 mg
Potassium: 51 mg

Exchange: 1 medium-fat meat

EGGPLANT RELISH ITALIANO ─────────────

Serve with bread or crackers as an appetizer, or try with pasta for an Italian entree.

1 eggplant (1½ pounds)
¼ cup olive oil
1½ cups thinly sliced celery
1 large onion, chopped
2 large red peppers, diced
3 cloves garlic, pressed

¼ cup (3 ounces) tomato paste
1 cup water
¼ cup red wine vinegar
1 tablespoon capers, drained
½ cup black olives, pitted and
   sliced

1. Cut unpeeled eggplant into ¼-inch cubes.
2. Warm oil in a 12- to 14-inch frying pan over medium heat. Add eggplant. Cover and cook until softened, about 5 minutes. Remove cover and continue cooking until eggplant is browned, about 10 minutes more.
3. Stir in celery, onion, peppers, and garlic. Cook until onion is soft.
4. Add the tomato paste, water, vinegar, capers, and olives.
5. Cook and stir mixture frequently until sauce is thick and eggplant is soft, about 10 minutes.
6. Serve cold or at room temperature. (This dish may be stored in the refrigerator up to 1 week.)

Yield: 12 servings, 3 cups
One Serving = ¼ cup

Calories: 73
Protein: 1 g
Fat: 5 g
Carbohydrate: 7 g

Fiber: 1.7 g
Cholesterol: 0
Sodium: 125 mg
Potassium: 242 mg

Exchange: 1 vegetable
          1 fat

GARLIC LOVER'S DIP _____ EASY

A different and interesting recipe! This dip is slightly higher in fat than some of our others. Serve with Toasted Pita Chips (p. 112) or No-Fry Tortilla Chips (p. 111).

> **2 cups prepared instant mashed potatoes (made without margarine or salt)**
> **6 medium cloves garlic, chopped**
> **½ teaspoon salt**
> **¼ cup olive oil**
> **¼ cup red wine vinegar**
> **2 tablespoons water**

1. In a food processor or blender, purée the mashed potatoes, garlic, and salt.
2. With machine running, gradually add oil, vinegar, and water and process until very smooth.
3. Cover and chill to allow flavors to blend for 1 to 2 hours before serving.

Yield: 6 servings, 1½ cups
One Serving = ¼ cup

Calories: 151	Fiber: 2.2 g
Protein: 3 g	Cholesterol: 0
Fat: 9 g	Sodium: 219 mg
Carbohydrate: 15 g	Potassium: 225 mg

Exchange: 1 starch/bread
           1½ fat

GUACAMOLE

We have modified this recipe to be lower in fat than the traditional version. Serve it with No-Fry Tortilla Chips (p. 111) or crunchy vegetables.

> 2 ounces tofu, cubed
> 3 green onions, chopped
> 2 ripe avocados, peeled, halved, pitted, and chopped
> 1 small tomato, diced
> 1 can (4 ounces) mild green chilies, drained and seeded
> 1 tablespoon freshly squeezed lemon juice
> 1 tablespoon Spicy Salsa (p. 109)
> 1 tablespoon chopped fresh cilantro
> ½ teaspoon cumin
> ⅛ teaspoon cayenne pepper
> Salt and freshly ground black pepper, to taste

1. In a blender or food processor, purée the tofu until smooth.
2. Add green onions, avocados, tomato, chilies, lemon juice, salsa, and seasonings.
3. Process until just blended; do not purée.

Yield: 8 servings, 2 cups
One Serving = ¼ cup

Calories: 94
Protein: 2 g
Fat: 8 g
Carbohydrate: 6 g

Fiber: 2.5 g
Cholesterol: 0
Sodium: 226 mg
Potassium: 381 mg

Exchange: 2 fat

PESTO DIP

Serve with Toasted Pita Chips (p. 112), low-fat crackers, or vegetables.

> 1½ cups fresh basil leaves, loosely packed
> 2 medium cloves garlic, minced
> 1 tablespoon olive oil
> ¼ cup freshly grated Parmesan cheese
> ½ cup low-fat cottage cheese
> 2 tablespoons freshly squeezed lemon juice
> Salt to taste
> 1 cherry tomato

1. Reserve 2 or 3 basil leaves for a garnish. Purée the remaining basil, garlic, and oil in a food processor or blender until smooth.
2. Add Parmesan and cottage cheeses, lemon juice, and salt, and blend until creamy.
3. Garnish before serving with reserved basil and a cherry tomato.

Yield: 6 servings, about 1½ cups
One Serving = ¼ cup

Calories: 69　　　　　Fiber: 1.2 g
Protein: 5 g　　　　　Cholesterol: 4 mg
Fat: 4 g　　　　　　　Sodium: 142 mg
Carbohydrate: 5 g　　Potassium: 223 mg

Exchange: 1 lean meat
　　　　　 1 vegetable

SALMON SPREAD

An elegant and easy appetizer. Serve with low-fat crackers or crispy vegetables.

> 1 can (15½ ounces) water-packed red salmon, drained
> 4 ounces part-skim ricotta cheese
> ½ tablespoon Tabasco sauce
> 1 tablespoon freshly squeezed lemon juice
> ½ teaspoon dill weed
> 1 tablespoon chopped fresh parsley

Combine ingredients thoroughly in a food processor or blender. Chill until serving time.

Yield: 16 servings, 2 cups
One Serving = 2 tablespoons

Calories: 48
Protein: 6 g
Fat: 2 g
Carbohydrate: <1 g

Fiber: trace
Cholesterol: 12 mg
Sodium: 165 mg
Potassium: 103 mg

Exchange: 1 lean meat

SPICY SALSA _____ EASY

1 can (16 ounces) whole tomatoes
1 small green pepper, chopped
⅓ cup chopped mild onion
3 tablespoons chopped green onion
1 can (4 ounces) diced green chilies, rinsed and drained
3 tablespoons chopped fresh cilantro
½ clove garlic, minced

1. Purée tomatoes with their juice in a blender or food processor.
2. Combine other ingredients and stir into tomatoes. (Chill in refrigerator up to 5 days.)

Yield: 7 servings, 2⅓ cups
One Serving = ⅓ cup

Calories: 21
Protein: <1 g
Fat: <1 g
Carbohydrate: 5 g

Fiber: 0.9 g
Cholesterol: 0
Sodium: 314 mg
Potassium: 192 mg

Exchange: 1 vegetable

TEMPEH PÂTÉ

Tempeh is a fermented soybean product that is seasoned and pressed. Look for it in health food stores or Asian markets. In this recipe, tempeh provides a tasty, low-fat alternative to meat pâtés — with no cholesterol! Spread on Toasted Pita Chips (p. 112) or Oat Bran Crackers (p. 182).

2 tablespoons margarine
½ package (4 ounces) tempeh, cubed
1 cup chopped onions
1 cup chopped mushrooms
2 cloves garlic, minced or pressed
1 tablespoon soy sauce
1 tablespoon dry sherry
½ teaspoon sage
⅛ teaspoon allspice

1. Melt margarine in a 10- to 12-inch skillet over medium-high heat.
2. Add tempeh, onions, mushrooms, and garlic, stirring often until onions begin to brown, about 5 minutes.
3. Stir in soy sauce, sherry, sage, and allspice.
4. Cook, stirring constantly, until all liquid is absorbed into the mixture. Remove from heat.
5. When cooled, pour into a food processor or blender and purée.
6. Pour into a bowl and chill for at least 1 hour before serving. (The pâté may be refrigerated for up to 3 days.)

Yield: 4 servings, 1 cup
One Serving = ¼ cup

Calories: 121
Protein: 11 g
Fat: 6 g
Carbohydrate: 6 g

Fiber: 1.1 g
Cholesterol: 0
Sodium: 265 mg
Potassium: 158 mg

Exchange: 1 lean meat
1 vegetable
1 fat

NO-FRY TORTILLA CHIPS

A delicious low-fat, low-sodium alternative to conventional corn chips. They go especially well with Guacamole (p. 107) and Spicy Salsa (p. 109).

1 package (12 ounces) or 12 corn tortillas, or 1 package (14 ounces) or 10 flour tortillas, 10-inch size

Salt (optional)

1. Immerse tortillas one at a time in water. Let drain briefly, then lay flat.

2. If desired, sprinkle tops lightly with salt.

3. Cut each tortilla into 6 to 8 wedges.

4. Cover a nonstick baking sheet with a single layer of tortilla wedges, salt side up. Place close together but do not overlap.

5. Bake in a 500°F oven for 4 minutes. Turn with a spatula; then continue to bake until golden brown and crisp, an additional 3 minutes for corn tortillas and 1 minute for flour tortillas. (Store in an airtight bag until ready to serve.)

Yield: 6 servings, 12 cups
One Serving = 2 cups, or 12 to 16 chips

	Corn tortilla chips	*Flour tortilla chips*
Calories	113	157
Protein	4 g	5 g
Fat	2 g	5 g
Carbohydrate	22 g	26 g
Fiber	1.7 g	3.26 g
Cholesterol	0	0
Sodium	90 mg	46 mg
Potassium	88 mg	136 mg

Exchange: 1½ starch/bread   Exchange: 1½ starch/bread
                                                      1 fat

PASTA CHIPS

1 package (16 ounces) lasagna noodles
2 teaspoons vegetable oil
¼ cup water
Nonstick vegetable spray
⅓ cup freshly grated Parmesan cheese
2 teaspoons basil
2 teaspoons oregano
2 teaspoons parsley flakes
¾ teaspoon garlic powder

1. Cook noodles according to package directions, omitting salt. Drain well. Separate noodles carefully on a flat surface.
2. Combine oil and water in a small bowl; stir well and brush both sides of lasagna noodles with the mixture. Cut each noodle crosswise into 2-inch pieces and arrange in a single layer on a baking sheet coated with cooking spray. Set aside.
3. Combine Parmesan cheese, basil, oregano, parsley, and garlic powder in a small bowl; stir well. Sprinkle a rounded ⅛ teaspoon of the herb mixture over each chip. Bake at 400°F for 16 minutes or until crisp and golden. Cool and store in an airtight container until ready to serve.

Yield: 24 servings, approximately 12 dozen chips
One Serving = 6 chips

Calories: 84	Fiber: 0.5 g
Protein: 3 g	Cholesterol: <1 mg
Fat: 1 g	Sodium: 24 mg
Carbohydrate: 16 g	Potassium: 48 mg

Exchange: 1 starch/bread

TOASTED PITA CHIPS

These are great with dips, soups, and in lunches. For more fiber, use whole wheat pita bread.

6 pita bread pockets
1 teaspoon garlic powder (optional)

1. Preheat oven to 325°F.
2. Split each pita pocket in half.
3. Cut each half into 6 triangles with a sharp knife.
4. Arrange in single layers on cookie sheets. Sprinkle lightly with garlic powder, if desired.
5. Bake for 8 minutes or until chips are lightly browned and very crisp. Store in an airtight container until ready to serve.

Yield: 8 cups or 64 chips
One Serving = 1 cup or 8 chips

Calories: 96	Fiber: 0.5 g
Protein: 3 g	Cholesterol: 0
Fat: <1 g	Sodium: 161 mg
Carbohydrate: 19 g	Potassium: 34 mg

Exchange: 1 starch/bread

CRAB MORNAY

An elegant filling for bite-size Cream Puffs (p. 282).

2 green onions, chopped
½ cup chopped mushrooms
¼ cup nonfat milk
1 teaspoon cornstarch
1 ounce low-fat Swiss cheese, freshly grated
½ cup imitation or fresh crabmeat

1. Sauté green onions and mushrooms in 2 tablespoons water until soft; set aside.
2. Combine milk and cornstarch, mixing well, and warm in a saucepan. Stir in vegetables, cooking until sauce is thickened.
3. Add cheese and crab; stir until cheese has melted.
4. Spoon into Cream Puff shells.
5. Serve warm or at room temperature.

Yield: 32 servings, 1 cup
One Serving = ½ tablespoon filling

Calories: 10	Fiber: trace
Protein: 1 g	Cholesterol: 1 mg
Fat: <1 g	Sodium: 28 mg
Carbohydrate: <1 g	Potassium: 14 mg

Exchange: 1 serving = free

SPICY SEAFOOD WONTONS ───────────────

A splash of Tabasco spices up these tasty appetizers.

4 ounces Neufchâtel cheese
1 cup imitation or fresh crabmeat
5 green onions, chopped
½ teaspoon Tabasco sauce
1 clove garlic, minced
25 wonton or pot sticker wrappers, or *gyoza* (round Japanese skins)
1 tablespoon vegetable oil
¼ cup water

1. Combine first 5 ingredients in food processor or blender until smooth.
2. Add 2 teaspoons of this filling to the middle of a wonton wrapper, fold in half over the mixture, and seal edges.
3. Heat oil in a large skillet over medium heat.
4. Place wontons in skillet and cook just until lightly browned on both sides.
5. Gradually pour water into skillet; cover immediately.
6. Allow to steam 1 minute.
7. Drain wontons with slotted spoon.
8. Serve immediately.

Yield: 12 servings, approximately 1 cup mixture, 24 wontons
One Serving = 2 wontons

Calories: 72	Fiber: <1 g
Protein: 4 g	Cholesterol: 38 mg
Fat: 4 g	Sodium: 42 mg
Carbohydrate: 4 g	Potassium: 40 mg

Exchange: 1 medium-fat meat

SPINACH APPETIZERS _____

1 package (10 ounces) frozen chopped spinach
½ cup fine bread crumbs
1 egg, lightly beaten
¼ cup part-skim ricotta cheese
¼ cup freshly grated Parmesan cheese
2 green onions, chopped
¼ teaspoon cumin
2 teaspoons freshly squeezed lemon juice

1. Preheat oven to 400°F.
2. Cook spinach according to package directions or just until tender.
3. Drain, and squeeze out excess water when cooled.
4. Stir in remaining ingredients and form mixture into 1-inch balls.
5. Place on a nonstick baking sheet and bake for 12 minutes or until lightly browned.

Yield: 5 servings, 15 appetizers
One Serving = 3 appetizers

Calories: 103	Fiber: 1.8 g
Protein: 7 g	Cholesterol: 62 mg
Fat: 4 g	Sodium: 211 mg
Carbohydrate: 11 g	Potassium: 179 mg

Exchange: ½ starch/bread
    1 vegetable
    ½ medium-fat meat

9

SOUPS AND SANDWICHES

SERVED HOT OR COLD, soups and sandwiches are the perfect combination. Our soup recipes feature fresh ingredients, including a wide selection of herbs and spices, and much less sodium than the canned variety. You can add almost any vegetable to a soup for more nutrition. Adding legumes and grains to a soup makes it heartier and more nutritious, as well. Increase the portion size and you have a satisfying entree. Keep in mind, however, that you may also be increasing your fat intake, so be sure to complement the soup with a crispy green salad, low-fat crackers, or a slice of fresh bread.

For sandwiches, you can spread several combinations of ingredients inside or atop breads, buns, tortillas, or bagels. Add crunchy vegetables like lettuce, tomatoes, sprouts, and cucumbers to increase volume without added calories and fat. Sandwiches are the perfect choice for the busy, on-the-go person. Be creative!

Creamy Mushroom Soup
French Onion Soup
Gazpacho
Hearty Lamb and Barley
    Stew
Lentil Soup
New England Soup
Simple Zucchini Soup
Sopa de Ajo (Garlic Soup)
Split Pea Soup
Tortilla Soup
White Bean Soup

Artichoke Pita Sandwiches
C-C-C Sandwich
California Chicken Sandwich
Chicken Tarragon Sandwich
Quick Pita Breakfast
Tuna Curry Sandwich
Turkey Club Sandwich

CREAMY MUSHROOM SOUP

1 tablespoon margarine
1½ cups coarsely chopped mushrooms
½ cup coarsely chopped onion
1 tablespoon all-purpose flour
2 cups low-fat milk
1 chicken bouillon cube
⅛ teaspoon nutmeg
⅛ teaspoon salt (optional)
⅛ teaspoon freshly ground black pepper (optional)

1. Melt margarine in a large saucepan.
2. Add mushrooms and onion, cooking until onion is soft.
3. Stir in flour, then remove from heat.
4. Gradually stir in milk, bouillon cube, and nutmeg.
5. Return to heat and cook, stirring constantly until thickened.
6. To thicken further, remove approximately 1½ cups of soup and blend until smooth in a blender or food processor. Return to the pot.
7. Add salt and pepper to taste, if desired.

Yield: 6 servings, 3 cups
One Serving = ½ cup

Calories: 76
Protein: 4 g
Fat: 4 g
Carbohydrate: 7 g

Fiber: 0.6 g
Cholesterol: 7 mg
Sodium: 181 mg (with salt)
Potassium: 239 mg

Exchange: 1 vegetable
          ½ low-fat milk

FRENCH ONION SOUP

    1 large onion, thinly sliced (about 1 cup)
    1 tablespoon margarine
    2 cans (10½ ounces each) condensed beef broth
    1½ cups water
    1 to 2 tablespoons dry sherry
    2 tablespoons Worcestershire sauce
    6 melba toast rounds
    6 teaspoons freshly grated low-fat cheese (part-skim mozzarella,
        Monterey Jack, or Swiss)

1. In a stockpot, cook the sliced onion in the margarine over low heat, about 5 minutes, or until onion is lightly browned.
2. Add the condensed beef broth, water, sherry, and Worcestershire sauce, and bring to a boil.
3. Pour the soup into 6 ovenproof cups.
4. Float a melba toast round on top of each bowl of soup; sprinkle each round with 1 teaspoon of grated cheese.
5. Broil 3 to 4 inches from heat for about 2 minutes or until browned.

Yield: 6 servings, 4½ cups
One Serving = ¾ cup

      Calories: 67   Fiber: 0.5 g
      Protein: 3 g   Cholesterol: 2 mg
      Fat: 3 g   Sodium: 389 mg
      Carbohydrate: 6 g   Potassium: 153 mg

Exchange: 1½ vegetable
           ½ fat

GAZPACHO ————————————————————————— EASY

Cold and refreshing, this soup is terrific during the hot summer months.

> **3 cups low-sodium tomato juice**
> **1 cup minced green pepper**
> **1 cucumber, diced (about 2 cups)**
> **2 green onions, chopped**
> **1 clove garlic, minced**
> **¼ cup chopped fresh parsley**
> **Dash of Tabasco sauce**
> **Freshly ground black pepper to taste**

1. Purée all ingredients in a blender or food processor.
2. Chill for at least 2 hours.
3. Serve cold or at room temperature.

Yield: 4 servings, 4 cups
One Serving = 1 cup

Calories: 48	Fiber: 3 g
Protein: 2 g	Cholesterol: 0
Fat: <1 g	Sodium: 23 mg
Carbohydrate: 11 g	Potassium: 402 mg

Exchange: 2 vegetable

HEARTY LAMB AND BARLEY STEW _____

  1 large onion, chopped
  1 clove garlic, minced
  ½ pound mushrooms
  1 pound lean lamb, trimmed and cubed (stew meat or sirloin end of leg)
  1 large parsnip, peeled and diced
  1 medium carrot, peeled and diced
  6 cups (or more) beef stock or canned low-sodium broth
  6 cups (or more) water
  1 bay leaf
  ½ cup medium pearl barley
  2 cups thinly sliced cabbage
  1 tablespoon tomato paste
  3 tablespoons chopped fresh parsley
  Salt and freshly ground black pepper (optional)

1. Combine onion and garlic in a large, heavy stockpot over very low heat. Cover and cook until onion is translucent and the edges start to brown, stirring occasionally, 20 to 30 minutes.
2. Thinly slice ¼ of the mushrooms and set aside. Finely chop the remaining mushrooms. Add chopped mushrooms, lamb, parsnip, carrot, stock, water, and a bay leaf to the pot and bring just to a boil, stirring frequently. Reduce heat; simmer 1 hour, stirring occasionally.
3. Stir barley into soup. Cover and simmer until barley is tender, about 30 minutes. Stir in sliced mushrooms, cabbage, and tomato paste, and simmer until vegetables are just tender, about 10 minutes. Add parsley. Season with salt and pepper, if desired. Remove bay leaf before serving.

Yield: 8 servings, about 8 to 10 cups
One Serving = 1 cup

Calories: 166	Fiber: 3.1 g
Protein: 13 g	Cholesterol: 33 mg
Fat: 5 g	Sodium: 125 mg
Carbohydrate: 17 g	Potassium: 491 mg

Exchange: ½ starch/bread
          1 medium-fat meat
          2 vegetable

LENTIL SOUP ———————————————————

The red lentils provide a pleasant change of color, but you can substitute brown lentils.

1 cup red lentils
2 stalks celery, chopped
4 cups vegetable stock or water
1 small potato, chopped
¼ cup chopped onion
¼ cup extra lean ham, chopped
2 bay leaves
¼ teaspoon freshly ground black
    pepper

Mix all ingredients in a stockpot and cook until the lentils are very soft, about 1 to 2 hours. Remove bay leaves and serve warm.

Yield: 4 servings, 4 cups
One Serving = 1 cup

Calories: 106
Protein: 7 g
Fat: 1 g
Carbohydrate: 18 g

Fiber: 4 g
Cholesterol: 5 mg
Sodium: 155 mg
Potassium: 386 mg

Exchange: 1 starch/bread
         ½ lean meat

NEW ENGLAND SOUP _____

A hearty soup for a chilly day. Serve with bread for a satisfying meal. Be sure to use the low-sodium canned tomato products or the salt content of the soup will be quite high.

1 onion, chopped
2 cloves garlic, minced
1 carrot, sliced
1 green pepper, diced
1 cup chopped broccoli
1 can (16 ounces) tomatoes, drained (low-sodium)
1 can (8 ounces) tomato sauce (low-sodium)
½ cup macaroni, uncooked
1 can (16 ounces) pinto beans
2 cups water
1 tablespoon oregano
1½ teaspoons freshly ground black pepper
1½ teaspoons basil

1. In a large nonstick pot, sauté onion and garlic until soft.
2. Stir in the remaining ingredients and cook until vegetables are tender and macaroni is cooked. Stir frequently.
3. Serve piping hot.

Yield: 6 servings, 6 cups
One Serving = 1 cup

Calories: 201
Protein: 11 g
Fat: 1 g
Carbohydrate: 39 g

Fiber: 10.5 g*
Cholesterol: 0
Sodium: 215 mg
Potassium: 938 mg

Exchange: 2 starch/bread
             2 vegetable

*Good source of dietary fiber

SIMPLE ZUCCHINI SOUP

1 pound zucchini, cut into 1-inch chunks
½ cup finely minced onion
1 teaspoon margarine
¼ teaspoon black pepper
¼ teaspoon basil
¼ teaspoon tarragon
¼ teaspoon thyme
1 teaspoon soy sauce
2 cups low-fat milk, heated but not scalding

1. Steam the zucchini until tender.
2. In a large saucepan, sauté the onion in the margarine.
3. Add the seasonings to the onion; stir in the zucchini.
4. Remove from heat and purée the vegetable mixture in a food processor or blender until smooth.
5. Return to the pan and slowly stir in the milk.
6. Cook over low heat until warm. Serve warm or cold.

Yield: 4 servings, 4 cups
One Serving = 1 cup

Calories: 94
Protein: 6 g
Fat: 4 g
Carbohydrate: 11 g

Fiber: 1.5 g
Cholesterol: 10 mg
Sodium: 162 mg
Potassium: 509 mg

Exchange: 1 vegetable
　　　　　½ low-fat milk

SOPA DE AJO (GARLIC SOUP) ————————————— EASY

Serve with a green garden salad sprinkled with fresh cilantro.

2 tablespoons minced garlic
1 tablespoon olive oil
1 cup whole wheat bread crumbs
4 cups Chicken Stock (p. 290)
½ teaspoon cayenne pepper
½ teaspoon paprika
2 tablespoons fresh chopped parsley (optional)

1. In a large saucepan, sauté garlic in oil until soft.
2. Stir in bread crumbs, stock, cayenne, and paprika.
3. Bring to a boil, then reduce heat and simmer for about 20 minutes, uncovered.
4. Garnish with parsley, if desired.

Yield: 4 servings, 4 cups
One Serving = 1 cup

Calories: 161	Fiber: 1 g
Protein: 6 g	Cholesterol: 1 mg
Fat: 6 g	Sodium: 242 mg
Carbohydrate: 22 g	Potassium: 201 mg

Exchange: 1½ bread
          1 fat

SPLIT PEA SOUP _____ EASY

This hearty soup can make a filling entree. Try it with a fresh green salad and Bread Sticks (p. 176).

½ cup chopped onion
1 tablespoon margarine
2 cups split peas
1 ham bone or 8 to 10 ounces lean ham chopped in large pieces
6 cups water
½ teaspoon salt (optional)
1 teaspoon basil
¼ teaspoon thyme
1 bay leaf

1. In a large stockpot, sauté onion in margarine until tender.
2. Add split peas, ham bone, and water.
3. Stir in seasonings.
4. Bring to a boil; then cover and simmer for about 1 hour.
5. Discard ham bone and bay leaf.
6. To thicken, remove 2 cups of soup (if you have used chopped lean ham, leave it in the pot) and purée in a blender until smooth.
7. Return puréed soup to the pot, stirring until blended.
8. Serve warm.

Yield: 8 servings, 8 cups
One Serving = 1 cup

Calories: 125
Protein: 11 g
Fat: 4 g
Carbohydrate: 11 g

Fiber: 2.7 g
Cholesterol: 17 mg
Sodium: 445 mg* (without salt)
Potassium: 316 mg

Exchange: 1 starch/bread
          1 lean meat

*High in sodium

TORTILLA SOUP

3 6-inch corn tortillas, cut into ½-inch strips
2 tomatoes
½ small onion, chopped
1 clove garlic, minced
½ green pepper, chopped
2 cups Chicken Stock (p. 290)
1 tablespoon chopped fresh cilantro
¼ cup freshly grated low-fat Monterey Jack cheese

1. Bake tortilla strips in the oven at 325°F for 5 to 7 minutes or until crisp.
2. Purée tomatoes, onion, garlic, and pepper in a food processor or blender.
3. Bring stock to a boil in a 2-quart pot. Stir in the tomato purée and cilantro.
4. Simmer on low heat for about 10 minutes.
5. Stir half of the tortilla strips into the soup.
6. Garnish with remaining tortilla strips and the cheese.

Yield: 6 servings, 3 cups
One Serving = ½ cup

Calories: 71	Fiber: 1.3 g
Protein: 4 g	Cholesterol: 5 mg
Fat: 3 g	Sodium: 313 mg
Carbohydrate: 9 g	Potassium: 210 mg

Exchange: ½ starch/bread
          1 vegetable

WHITE BEAN SOUP

3 to 4 cloves garlic, crushed
1 cup chopped onion
1 tablespoon olive oil
1 carrot, chopped
1 stalk celery, chopped
4 cups vegetable stock or water
¼ cup dry white wine
2 cups cooked (1 cup raw) white beans
½ cup black olives, pitted and sliced
1 tablespoon freshly squeezed lemon juice
2 teaspoons tarragon
Salt and freshly ground black pepper (optional)

1. In a large stockpot, sauté garlic and onion in oil.
2. Stir in carrot and celery.
3. Add stock, wine, cooked beans, olives, lemon juice, and seasonings.
4. Cover and simmer for 30 to 45 minutes.
5. Serve hot.

Yield: 6 servings, 6 cups
One Serving = 1 cup

Calories: 139
Protein: 6 g
Fat: 4 g
Carbohydrate: 20 g

Fiber: 6.9 g*
Cholesterol: 0
Sodium: 166 mg (with salt)
Potassium: 447 mg

Exchange: 1 starch/bread
1 vegetable
½ lean meat

*Good source of dietary fiber

ARTICHOKE PITA SANDWICHES ——————————— QUICK

Filling

    4 ounces canned or frozen artichoke hearts
    1 ounce feta cheese, crumbled
    2 green onions, minced
    1 small tomato, diced
    1 teaspoon olive oil
    2 teaspoons red wine vinegar
    1 teaspoon basil
    1 teaspoon chopped fresh parsley

    1 6-inch pita bread pocket, sliced in half
    Lettuce leaves
    Alfalfa sprouts (optional)

1. Drain canned artichoke hearts or thaw frozen artichoke hearts, and chop.
2. Combine all filling ingredients and stir well.
3. Stuff lettuce leaves in bread. Spoon ½ cup filling into each pita half and top with alfalfa sprouts, if desired.

Yield: 2 servings, 1 cup filling
One Serving = ½ cup filling, ½ pita bread pocket

    Calories: 214   Fiber: 6.5 g*
    Protein: 8 g   Cholesterol: 13 mg
    Fat: 6 g   Sodium: 438 mg†
    Carbohydrate: 33 g   Potassium: 364 mg

Exchange: 1½ starch/bread
           ½ high-fat meat
           2 vegetable

*Good source of dietary fiber
†High in sodium

C-C-C SANDWICH _____ EASY

Serve with a crispy salad or low-fat soup.

> **4 ounces Neufchâtel cheese, softened**
> **2 carrots, grated**
> **8 slices whole wheat bread**
> **½ medium cucumber, sliced**
> **4 teaspoons raw sunflower seeds, unsalted**
> **1 cup alfalfa sprouts**

1. Mix cheese with carrots in a bowl.
2. Spread 2 tablespoons of the mixture evenly on 4 slices of whole wheat bread.
3. Place 4 cucumber slices on top of cheese mixture and sprinkle with 1 teaspoon sunflower seeds.
4. Top with sprouts and a second slice of bread.

Yield: 4 sandwiches
One Serving = 1 sandwich

Calories: 251	Fiber: 5.1 g*
Protein: 10 g	Cholesterol: 23 mg
Fat: 10 g	Sodium: 428 mg†
Carbohydrate: 33 g	Potassium: 373 mg

Exchange: 2 starch/bread
              1 medium-fat meat
              ½ fat

*Good source of dietary fiber
†High in sodium

CALIFORNIA CHICKEN SANDWICH —————— MICROWAVE

A delicious use for last night's chicken. Grill, rather than broil, for a summertime cookout.

> 2 3-ounce boneless chicken breasts, cut into thin strips
> 6 asparagus spears
> 4 tablespoons finely grated Cheddar cheese
> 4 teaspoons plain nonfat yogurt
> 2 teaspoons Dijon-style mustard
> ½ teaspoon freshly squeezed lemon juice
> Lettuce leaves
> 2 slices sourdough bread
> Sun-dried tomatoes (optional)

1. Cook chicken strips in microwave on high for 5 to 7 minutes.
2. Cook asparagus spears in microwave on high for 4 to 5 minutes or until crisp-tender.
3. Meanwhile, combine cheese, yogurt, mustard, and lemon juice in a small bowl.
4. Place lettuce leaves on one slice of bread.
5. Arrange chicken strips and asparagus on top in an alternating pattern.
6. Pour cheese sauce over sandwich.
7. Top with sun-dried tomatoes, if desired.
8. Broil to warm sandwich and melt cheese until golden brown, about 5 minutes.

Yield: 2 open-faced sandwiches
One Serving = 1 sandwich

Calories: 218	Fiber: 0.8 g
Protein: 21 g	Cholesterol: 51 mg
Fat: 7 g	Sodium: 351 mg
Carbohydrate: 17 g	Potassium: 334 mg

Exchange: 1 starch/bread
           2 lean meat
           1 vegetable

CHICKEN TARRAGON SANDWICH ——————— EASY

Serve this mixture over a bagel half with crispy lettuce and sliced tomato.

2 cups cooked chicken, cubed
¾ cup sliced celery
¼ cup chopped green onions or chives
½ cup plain low-fat yogurt
2 tablespoons reduced-calorie mayonnaise
1½ teaspoons tarragon
4 teaspoons slivered almonds, toasted
Salt and freshly ground black pepper

1. In a large bowl, combine chicken, celery, onions, yogurt, mayonnaise, and tarragon. Mix lightly.
2. Cover and refrigerate up to 24 hours.
3. Toss with almonds. Add salt and pepper to taste.

Yield: 6 servings, 3 cups
One Serving = ½ cup

Calories: 106
Protein: 13 g
Fat: 4 g
Carbohydrate: 3 g

Fiber: 0.5 g
Cholesterol: 37 mg
Sodium: 136 mg
Potassium: 218 mg

Exchange: 1½ lean meat
        1 vegetable

QUICK PITA BREAKFAST _____ EASY

A healthful, sandwich-style breakfast idea. Also great for a brown bag lunch.

1 small apple, diced
¼ cup low-fat cottage cheese
1 tablespoon raisins
½ whole wheat pita bread pocket

1. Combine apple, cottage cheese, and raisins.
2. Fill pita pocket with mixture.

Yield: 1 serving, 1 sandwich
One Serving = 1 sandwich

Calories: 223
Protein: 11 g
Fat: 2 g
Carbohydrate: 43 g

Fiber: 5.6 g*
Cholesterol: 5 mg
Sodium: 361 mg
Potassium: 334 mg

Exchange: 1 starch/bread
         ½ lean meat
         2 fruit

*Good source dietary fiber

TUNA CURRY SANDWICH ————————————— EASY

¼ cup reduced-calorie mayonnaise
½ teaspoon curry powder
1 can (6½ ounces) chunk-style, water-packed tuna, drained
¾ cup (1 medium) apple, chopped
2 tablespoons raisins
½ cup finely chopped celery
2 tablespoons thinly sliced green onion
4 slices raisin or whole wheat bread

1. Mix together mayonnaise and curry powder.
2. Stir in tuna, apple, raisins, celery, and onion until blended.
3. Toast bread and spread equal portions of tuna mixture over each slice.

Yield: 4 open-faced sandwiches
One Serving = 1 sandwich

Calories: 217
Protein: 16 g
Fat: 6 g
Carbohydrate: 28 g

Fiber: 3.5 g
Cholesterol: 22 mg
Sodium: 400 mg
Potassium: 371 mg

Exchange: 1 starch/bread
1 lean meat
1 fruit
½ fat

TURKEY CLUB SANDWICH

A special treat for hearty appetites. The Cheesy Herb Spread lends a subtle, tangy taste to this sandwich.

> **12 slices raisin bread**
> **Cheesy Herb Spread**
> **4 large tomato slices (1 tomato)**
> **8 slices cooked turkey (about ½ ounce each)**
> **1 cup alfalfa sprouts**

Cheesy Herb Spread
> **6-ounce package Neufchâtel cheese, softened**
> **2 tablespoons chopped fresh parsley**
> **½ teaspoon dry mustard**
> **1 tablespoon chopped onion**
> **Salt and freshly ground black pepper**
> **Dash of garlic powder**

1. Combine all the ingredients for the Cheesy Herb Spread in a small bowl. Season to taste.
2. For each sandwich, spread 1 slice raisin bread with 2 tablespoons of the cheese mixture.
3. Top with tomato slice sandwiched between 2 slices of turkey.
4. Place a second slice of bread on top.
5. Spread the remaining 4 slices of bread with 2 tablespoons more of Cheesy Herb Spread and sprouts, and add a third layer to each sandwich.
6. Cut each sandwich into 4 triangles and secure with toothpicks, if desired.

Yield: 4 sandwiches
One Serving = 1 sandwich

Calories: 362	Fiber: 2.5 g
Protein: 18 g	Cholesterol: 45 mg
Fat: 14 g	Sodium: 924 mg*
Carbohydrate: 43 g	Potassium: 394 mg

Exchange: 3 starch/bread
          2 medium-fat meat
          1 fat

*High in sodium

10
SALADS AND DRESSINGS

SALADS OFFER more exciting variety, color, and flavor than almost any other group of foods. Our recipes feature a wide variety of high-fiber vegetables, pastas, and beans combined in new and different ways. Some of the marinated salads, such as those containing white beans and pinto beans, are relatively high in calories and fat (10 grams or 2 teaspoons per serving). You should eat them less frequently than green salads or some of the pasta salads with low-fat dressings. However, they are high in soluble fiber and offer new ways to incorporate legumes into the diet. We recommend eating the marinated salads no more than 2 to 3 times per week. They make a nice light main dish or lunch along with nonfat yogurt, skim-milk cheese, or low-fat cottage cheese.

Regular salad dressings are high in fat, which accounts for almost 90 percent of their total calories. We offer some lower-fat alternatives, but you should always use dressings sparingly. Complement the meal with other sources of complex carbohydrate, such as whole grain rolls or freshly baked bread.

Basil and Tomato Salad	Red Pepper and Broccoli Salad
Citrus Salad	Shrimp and Pasta Salad
Fiesta Bean Salad	Spinach Salad
Fruit Strata Salad	Summer Salad
Gazpacho Salad	Sunny Salad
Greek Pasta Salad	Sweet and Sour Cabbage Salad
Marinated White Bean Salad	
Picnic Potato Salad	

Tabbouli

Watermelon Salad with
Raspberry Vinegar

Low-Fat Creamy Garlic
Dressing

Low-Fat Thousand Island
Dressing

Sprout Dressing

Traditional Vinaigrette
Dressing

BASIL AND TOMATO SALAD ——————————— EASY

A great accompaniment to any fresh pasta dish.

3 small tomatoes, diced
¼ cup chopped fresh basil leaves
2 teaspoons olive oil
1 tablespoon white vinegar
½ cup diced part-skim mozzarella cheese

1. Mix tomatoes and basil in a large salad bowl. Toss in oil, vinegar, and cheese; blend thoroughly.
2. Let the salad stand for 10 minutes before serving.
3. Serve at room temperature.

Yield: 4 servings, 2 cups
One Serving = ½ cup

Calories: 94
Protein: 6 g
Fat: 6 g
Carbohydrate: 6 g

Fiber: 2 g
Cholesterol: 10 mg
Sodium: 100 mg
Potassium: 306 mg

Exchange: 1 medium-fat meat
1 vegetable

CITRUS SALAD ————————————————————— EASY

> **1 large pink grapefruit, peeled and cut into chunks**
> **1 large orange, peeled and cut into chunks**
> **1 stalk celery, chopped**
> **1 tablespoon chopped walnuts**
> **½ avocado, peeled, pitted, and cut into chunks**
> **Lettuce leaf**

1. Combine all ingredients.
2. Serve on a dark green lettuce leaf.

Yield: 4 servings, 4 cups
One Serving = 1 cup

Calories: 109	Fiber: 3.2 g
Protein: 2 g	Cholesterol: 0
Fat: 5 g	Sodium: 11 mg
Carbohydrate: 16 g	Potassium: 415 mg

Exchange: 1 fruit
           1 fat

FIESTA BEAN SALAD

Accompany this salad with Tortilla Soup (p. 126) and No-Fry Tortilla Chips (p. 111) and you have a meal — appropriate for lunch or a light supper.

1 can (15 ounces) red kidney beans
1 can (15 ounces) pinto beans
1 can (5 ounces) whole kernel corn
½ cup thinly sliced green onion
¼ cup chopped fresh parsley
1 cup sliced celery
1 can (4 ounces) green chilies, diced
¼ cup vegetable oil
¼ cup cider or wine vinegar
1 to 2 cloves garlic, minced
1 teaspoon chili powder
1 teaspoon oregano
¼ teaspoon cumin
¼ to ½ teaspoon freshly ground black pepper or taco sauce

1. Drain and rinse beans and corn.
2. Combine beans and corn with the green onion, parsley, celery, and chilies in a bowl.
3. In a separate bowl, mix together the oil, vinegar, and seasonings.
4. Pour dressing over salad and mix well.
5. Chill 2 hours or overnight.
6. Before serving, stir several times to blend flavors.

Yield: 8 servings, 8 cups
One Serving = 1 cup

Calories: 190	Fiber: 8.6 g*
Protein: 8 g	Cholesterol: 0
Fat: 7 g	Sodium: 374 mg
Carbohydrate: 25 g	Potassium: 569 mg

Exchange: 1½ starch/bread
1 medium-fat meat

*Good source of dietary fiber

FRUIT STRATA SALAD _____

> 3 cups torn green leaf lettuce
> 1 honeydew melon, peeled and cubed
> 1 pint strawberries, hulled and halved
> 1 can (20 ounces) pineapple chunks in their own juice, drained
> 1 large banana, sliced
> 1 cup low- or nonfat lemon or vanilla yogurt
> 2 ounces freshly grated low-fat Swiss cheese
> ¼ cup fresh mint leaves

1. Place half the lettuce in a large salad bowl.
2. Layer fruits on top of the lettuce, reserving 8 strawberry halves for garnish. Top with remaining lettuce.
3. Spread yogurt over top; sprinkle with grated cheese.
4. Cover and chill 2 to 3 hours.
5. Garnish with reserved strawberry halves and fresh mint.
6. Toss gently to serve.

Yield: 12 servings, 12 cups
One Serving = 1 cup

Calories: 95
Protein: 3 g
Fat: <1 g
Carbohydrate: 21 g

Fiber: 1.8 g
Cholesterol: 3 mg
Sodium: 87 mg
Potassium: 355 mg

Exchange: 1 fruit
         ½ low-fat milk

GAZPACHO SALAD _____

Instead of blending the vegetables to make the traditional soup, stop at the chopping phase, and serve as a salad.

    1 medium tomato, chopped
    ½ medium cucumber, chopped
    ½ medium green pepper, seeded and chopped
    1 stalk celery, finely chopped
    ¼ cup chopped onion
    1 tablespoon chopped fresh parsley

Herb Dressing
    3 tablespoons red wine vinegar
    2 tablespoons freshly squeezed lemon juice
    1 tablespoon olive oil
    1 teaspoon Dijon-style mustard
    ½ teaspoon oregano
    ½ teaspoon garlic powder

    Lettuce leaves

1. Combine first 6 ingredients in a 13 × 9 × 2-inch baking dish.
2. Combine all ingredients for the Herb Dressing and mix or whisk until thoroughly blended.
3. Pour dressing over the vegetables; toss gently.
4. Chill at least 2 hours.
5. Arrange lettuce leaves on serving platter. Spoon salad over leaves and serve.

Yield for salad: 5 servings
One Serving = ½ cup

Yield for dressing: ½ cup
One Serving = 1½ to 2 tablespoons

    Calories: 57   Fiber: 2.8 g
    Protein: 2 g   Cholesterol: 0
    Fat: 3 g   Sodium: 34 mg
    Carbohydrate: 7 g   Potassium: 335 mg

Exchange: 1 vegetable
        ½ fat

GREEK PASTA SALAD

¼ pound (1 cup) fresh green beans, trimmed and halved
2 cups corkscrew pasta (rotini), cooked according to package directions
2 cups cubed poached chicken breasts
1 cup canned or frozen artichoke hearts, drained and chopped
1 ounce crumbled feta cheese
1 tomato, chopped

Dressing

2 tablespoons olive oil
¼ cup freshly squeezed lemon juice
2 teaspoons red wine vinegar
1 teaspoon basil
¼ teaspoon oregano
2 cloves garlic, finely chopped
Salt and freshly ground black pepper to taste

1. Steam green beans and cook until crisp-tender, about 5 minutes. Drain in a colander and rinse with cold water.
2. In a large bowl, combine beans with the rest of the salad ingredients.
3. In a small bowl, whisk together the dressing ingredients and pour over the salad. Mix thoroughly. Adjust seasonings to taste.
4. Serve at once, or refrigerate, covered, until serving time.

Yield: 6 servings, 6 cups
One Serving = 1 cup

Calories: 225
Protein: 19 g
Fat: 8 g
Carbohydrate: 19 g

Fiber: 2.6 g
Cholesterol: 57 mg
Sodium: 344 mg
Potassium: 340 mg

Exchange: 1 bread
2 lean meat
1 vegetable

MARINATED WHITE BEAN SALAD _____

**2 pounds white beans, soaked, cooked according to package directions
    until tender, and rinsed under cold water**
¼ cup olive oil
¼ cup freshly squeezed lemon juice
2 tablespoons freshly squeezed orange juice
½ cup chopped red onion
1 tablespoon minced garlic
½ cup chopped tomatoes
¼ cup black olives, pitted and diced
1½ teaspoons oregano
¼ cup chopped fresh parsley
Salt and freshly ground black pepper to taste

1. Combine beans with olive oil, lemon juice, and orange juice.
2. Add onion, garlic, tomatoes, olives, and oregano. Toss thoroughly.
3. Add parsley and salt and pepper to taste.
4. Marinate at least 3 hours before serving.

Yield: 8 servings, 6 cups
One Serving = ¾ cup

Calories: 233	Fiber: 6.2 g*
Protein: 12 g	Cholesterol: 0
Fat: 4 g	Sodium: 96 mg
Carbohydrate: 37 g	Potassium: 841 mg

Exchange: 2 starch/bread
          1 lean meat
          1 vegetable

*Good source of dietary fiber

PICNIC POTATO SALAD _____

4 red potatoes
¼ cup plain nonfat yogurt
2 tablespoons reduced-calorie mayonnaise
2 teaspoons Dijon-style mustard
1 cup chopped celery
1 red onion, chopped
2 teaspoons celery seeds

1. Steam or boil potatoes until just tender.
2. Drain and refrigerate until chilled.
3. Combine yogurt, mayonnaise, and mustard. Mix well.
4. Dice potatoes, add celery and onion, and toss with yogurt mixture.
5. Sprinkle with celery seeds.

Yield: 6 servings, 3 cups
One Serving = ½ cup

Calories: 122
Protein: 3 g
Fat: 2 g
Carbohydrate: 24 g

Fiber: 2.8 g
Cholesterol: 2 mg
Sodium: 83 mg
Potassium: 464 mg

Exchange: 1½ starch/bread

RED PEPPER AND BROCCOLI SALAD _____

1 large bunch of broccoli (approximately 2 cups), trimmed and cut into florets, stems peeled and cut on the diagonal

½ cup seeded and coarsely chopped red peppers

Creamy Cheese Dressing
½ cup low-fat cottage cheese
¼ cup chopped fresh parsley
⅛ cup reduced-calorie mayonnaise
1 green onion, minced
1 tablespoon freshly squeezed lemon juice
1 tablespoon skim milk
1 teaspoon Dijon-style mustard

1. Steam broccoli and peppers until crisp. Refrigerate until cooled.
2. Arrange broccoli and peppers in a large, shallow serving bowl or on a platter lined with lettuce leaves. Set aside.
3. Place all dressing ingredients in a blender or food processor.
4. Blend 30 seconds or until smooth, scraping sides of container as necessary.
5. Cover and chill.
6. Before serving, toss vegetables with Creamy Cheese Dressing.

Yield for salad: 5 servings, 2½ cups
One Serving = ½ cup

Yield for dressing: 5 servings, ¾ cup
One Serving = 1 tablespoon

Calories: 53	Fiber: 1.5 g
Protein: 5 g	Cholesterol: 4 mg
Fat: 2 g	Sodium: 118 mg
Carbohydrate: 6 g	Potassium: 195 mg

Exchange: 1 vegetable
         ½ fat

SHRIMP AND PASTA SALAD

¼ cup plain low-fat yogurt
1 tablespoon reduced-calorie mayonnaise
1 teaspoon Dijon-style mustard
¼ teaspoon dill weed
¼ teaspoon sweet basil
3 cups cooked rigatoni
6 ounces small shrimp, shelled, deveined, and cooked
½ cup green peas, steamed
¼ cup chopped red pepper
2 green onions, chopped

1. Blend yogurt, mayonnaise, mustard, dill weed, and basil; stir until smooth.
2. Mix noodles, shrimp, peas, pepper, and onion in a bowl.
3. Stir yogurt mixture into noodle mixture and refrigerate 2 to 4 hours before serving.

Yield: 4 servings, 4 cups
One Serving = 1 cup

Calories: 233
Protein: 16 g
Fat: 4 g
Carbohydrate: 33 g

Fiber: 2.3 g
Cholesterol: 122 mg
Sodium: 165 mg
Potassium: 239 mg

Exchange: 2 starch/bread
1 lean meat
½ fat

SPINACH SALAD _____

½ pound torn fresh spinach
2 teaspoons unsalted sunflower
    seeds
1 carrot, thinly sliced

½ green pepper, chopped
8 ounces water chestnuts, sliced
2 tablespoons freshly grated
    Parmesan cheese

1. Thoroughly wash and drain spinach.
2. Add sunflower seeds, carrot, green pepper, and water chestnuts to spinach in a bowl.
3. Toss with Traditional Vinaigrette Dressing (p. 153).
4. Top with Parmesan cheese.

Yield: 4 servings, 4 cups
One Serving = 1 cup

Calories: 79
Protein: 5 g
Fat: 2 g
Carbohydrate: 13 g

Fiber: 4.6 g
Cholesterol: 2 mg
Sodium: 200 mg
Potassium: 595 mg

Exchange: 2 vegetable
        ½ fat

SUMMER SALAD _____

½ cantaloupe, peeled and cubed
1 cup hulled and halved strawberries
1 cup halved green seedless grapes
1 apple, cored and chopped
½ cup evaporated skim milk, chilled
⅓ cup frozen orange juice concentrate, unsweetened, partially thawed
    (3-ounce can)
Lettuce leaves

1. Combine fruit and mix well.
2. Blend evaporated milk with orange juice; pour over fruit to coat.
3. Serve on lettuce-lined plates.

Yield: 8 servings, 6 cups
One Serving = ¾ cup

Calories: 56	Fiber: 1.3 g
Protein: 2 g	Cholesterol: <1 mg
Fat: <1 g	Sodium: 11 mg
Carbohydrate: 13 g	Potassium: 217 mg

Exchange: 1 fruit

SUNNY SALAD ─────────────────────────── QUICK

2 tablespoons raw sunflower seeds, unsalted
2 heads Boston or butterhead lettuce, torn into small pieces
2 cups sliced mushrooms
2 cups alfalfa sprouts
1 cup mung bean sprouts
2 tablespoons raisins
1 tomato, sliced
½ avocado, peeled and cubed

1. Combine all ingredients and toss.
2. Serve with Low-Fat Thousand Island Dressing (p. 151).

Yield: 6 servings, 6 cups
One Serving = 1 cup

Calories: 83	Fiber: 3.5 g
Protein: 3 g	Cholesterol: 0
Fat: 4 g	Sodium: 13 mg
Carbohydrate: 10 g	Potassium: 392 mg

Exchange: 2 vegetable
           1 fat

SWEET AND SOUR CABBAGE SALAD _____

    2 cups shredded green cabbage
    1 cup shredded red cabbage
    2 green onions, thinly sliced
    ¼ cup chopped fresh parsley
    ½ cup thinly sliced celery
    ⅓ cup thinly sliced green pepper

Dressing
    1 teaspoon Equal (3 packages)
    3 tablespoons white vinegar
    2 tablespoons vegetable oil
    ½ teaspoon salt

1. Combine vegetables in a bowl and chill.
2. Combine dressing ingredients and chill.
3. Just before serving, pour vinegar dressing over the vegetables and toss lightly.

Yield: 6 servings, 4 cups
One Serving = ⅔ cup

Calories: 66
Protein: <1 g
Fat: 6 g
Carbohydrate: 5 g

Fiber: 2 g
Cholesterol: 0
Sodium: 222 mg
Potassium: 221 mg

Exchange: 1 vegetable
        1 fat

TABBOULI

A traditional Middle Eastern dish containing bulgur wheat and fresh herbs. Serve with Toasted Pita Chips (p. 112) and raw vegetables.

1 cup bulgur wheat
2 cups boiling water
2 tomatoes, finely diced
1 bunch green onions, sliced
3 tablespoons chopped fresh mint, or 2 teaspoons dried
2 cups finely chopped fresh parsley
½ cup freshly squeezed lemon juice
¼ cup olive oil
Freshly ground black pepper to taste

1. Place uncooked bulgur in a bowl; pour boiling water over it and let it soak 1 hour (stir occasionally).
2. Drain well in a fine strainer.
3. Return bulgur to the bowl and add all other ingredients; mix well.
4. Chill for 2 hours.

Yield: 8 servings, 6 cups
One Serving = ¾ cup

Calories: 179
Protein: 4 g
Fat: 7 g
Carbohydrate: 26 g

Fiber: 0.3 g
Cholesterol: 0
Sodium: 9 mg
Potassium: 254 mg

Exchange: 1 starch/bread
2 vegetable
1 fat

WATERMELON SALAD WITH RASPBERRY VINEGAR — EASY

A deliciously different salad — it actually absorbs only a small amount of oil.

3 to 4 cups cubed watermelon
1 large red onion, thinly sliced

Vinaigrette
½ cup raspberry vinegar
Freshly ground black pepper to taste
½ cup vegetable oil
1 teaspoon low-fat vanilla yogurt

1. Mix melon and onion together and let marinate in a colander for at least 1 hour.
2. Combine vinegar and pepper; gradually whisk in oil.
3. Adjust seasoning and add yogurt. Stir in melon and onion.
4. Serve immediately.

Yield: 8 servings, 4 cups
One Serving = ½ cup

Calories: 72	Fiber: 0.6 g
Protein: 1 g	Cholesterol: 0
Fat: 5 g	Sodium: 2 mg
Carbohydrate: 6 g	Potassium: 130 mg

Exchange: ½ fruit
         1 fat

LOW-FAT CREAMY GARLIC DRESSING ——————— QUICK

This original, low-calorie recipe is equally good as a dip or dolloped on crisp hearts of lettuce.

4 large cloves garlic, finely minced
1 cup plain nonfat yogurt
½ cup reduced-calorie mayonnaise
½ teaspoon Dijon-style mustard

Combine all ingredients and chill until ready to use.

Yield: 12 servings, 1½ cups
One Serving = 2 tablespoons

Calories: 45
Protein: 1 g
Fat: 4 g
Carbohydrate: 3 g

Fiber: trace
Cholesterol: 7 mg
Sodium: 99 mg
Potassium: 53 mg

Exchange: 1 fat

LOW-FAT THOUSAND ISLAND DRESSING —————— QUICK

½ cup low-fat cottage cheese
2 tablespoons plain nonfat yogurt
2 tablespoons reduced-calorie mayonnaise or 1 tablespoon regular
  mayonnaise
2 tablespoons catsup
1 tablespoon nonfat milk (or more for a thinner consistency)
Dash of cayenne pepper
1 tablespoon pickle relish
1 tablespoon chopped onion

1. Thoroughly blend the first 6 ingredients.
2. Stir in pickle relish and onion.

Yield: 16 servings, 1 cup
One Serving = 1 tablespoon

Calories: 17
Protein: 1 g
Fat: <1 g
Carbohydrate: 2 g

Fiber: 0
Cholesterol: 1 mg
Sodium: 70 mg
Potassium: 24 mg

Exchange: 1 tablespoon = free
          2 to 3 tablespoons = 1 fat

When your sprouts begin to wilt, you can still put their flavor and nutrients to good use in this salad dressing.

1½ cups alfalfa sprouts
2 tablespoons red wine vinegar
½ cup safflower oil
1 package Equal
½ teaspoon parsley
½ teaspoon freshly ground black pepper
⅛ teaspoon garlic powder
1 tablespoon chopped green onion

1. Combine ingredients in a blender or food processor until smooth, about 1 minute.
2. Serve over salad.

Yield: 24 servings, 1½ cups
One Serving = 1 tablespoon

Calories: 41
Protein: <1 g
Fat: 5 g
Carbohydrate: <1 g

Fiber: 0.1 g
Cholesterol: 0
Sodium: <1 mg
Potassium: 5 mg

Exchange: 1 fat

TRADITIONAL VINAIGRETTE DRESSING ———————— QUICK

This traditional vinaigrette will enhance the taste of any salad. Try the low-fat version that follows to cut fat and calorie content in half.

¼ cup red wine vinegar or raspberry vinegar
1 small clove garlic, minced
¼ teaspoon salt
¼ teaspoon freshly ground black pepper
½ teaspoon Dijon-style mustard
½ cup olive oil

1. Combine all ingredients except oil in a medium bowl or food processor; blend well.
2. Slowly add oil in a stream, mixing until thickened. (The dressing will keep 1 to 2 weeks in the refrigerator.)

Yield: 12 servings, ¾ cup
One Serving = 1 tablespoon

Calories: 88   Fiber: 0
Protein: 0   Cholesterol: 0
Fat: 10 g   Sodium: 51 mg
Carbohydrate: <1 g   Potassium: 7 mg

Exchange: 2 fat

Low-Fat Version
Reduce oil to ¼ cup and add ¼ cup water.

One Serving = 1 tablespoon

Calories: 44   Fiber: 0
Protein: 0   Cholesterol: 0
Fat: 5 g   Sodium: 46 mg
Carbohydrate: <1 g   Potassium: 7 mg

Exchange: 1 fat

11

VEGETABLES AND SIDE DISHES

TRADITIONALLY used to accompany the main course, these side dishes and vegetable recipes make wonderful meatless entrees if you simply increase the portion sizes. Stuffed Tomatoes, Zucchini Boats, and Stir-fried Vegetables are just three examples.

Quick preparation by steaming, microwave cooking, or stir-frying retains flavor and nutritive value (fiber, vitamins, and minerals). Avoid adding excessive amounts of butter, margarine, mayonnaise, or creamy sauces to your vegetables. Instead, add zest by sprinkling them with lemon juice, herb vinegars, chili powder, hot sauce, or a tablespoon of Parmesan cheese.

Baked Stuffed Potatoes	Mediterranean Vegetables
Black Forest Mushrooms	Popeye's Favorite Spinach
Cauliflower Curry	Red Cabbage with Apples
Confetti Corn	Stir-fried Vegetables
German Potato Bake	Stuffed Acorn Squash
Ginger-Lemon Broccoli	Stuffed Green Peppers
Green Beans and Mustard Vinaigrette	Stuffed Tomatoes
Italian Vegetables	Zucchini Boats
Marinated Cucumbers	

BAKED STUFFED POTATOES

These stuffed potatoes are delicious cold or reheated. Eat leftovers for lunch the following day. Pair with a small salad or a cup of soup.

2 large potatoes
½ cup broccoli florets
⅓ cup plain nonfat yogurt
1 tablespoon nonfat milk
2 tablespoons freshly grated Parmesan cheese
2 tablespoons crumbled Roquefort or blue cheese
1 tablespoon low-fat cottage cheese
2 teaspoons basil
¼ teaspoon garlic powder

1. Wash potatoes, pat dry, and pierce with a knife.
2. Bake in a 375°F oven for 70 minutes or until done.
3. While potatoes are baking, steam broccoli until tender; set aside.
4. Cut potatoes in half lengthwise and carefully scoop out inside. Set skins aside.
5. Mash potato with a fork. Add yogurt, milk, cheeses, basil, and garlic powder. Beat until fluffy.
6. Gently stir in broccoli florets until mixture is well blended.
7. Carefully spoon mixture back into potato skins and return to the oven. Bake until heated through or place under broiler to brown tops.

Yield: 4 servings, 2 potatoes
One Serving = ½ potato with filling

Calories: 173
Protein: 8 g
Fat: 3 g
Carbohydrate: 29 g

Fiber: 3.6 g
Cholesterol: 9 mg
Sodium: 203 mg
Potassium: 594 mg

Exchange: 1 starch/bread
1 vegetable
½ low-fat milk

BLACK FOREST MUSHROOMS ───────────────

Great with grilled food! This is a very flavorful side dish.

   ½ cup chopped onion
   2 teaspoons olive oil
   2 cups sliced fresh mushrooms
   ½ cup chopped green peppers

Sauce
   2 tablespoons Dijon-style mustard
   2 tablespoons Worcestershire sauce
   1 teaspoon molasses
   2 tablespoons sherry
   Freshly ground black pepper to taste

1. Sauté onion in oil until transparent.
2. Add mushrooms and green pepper to onion, stirring often.
3. Combine sauce ingredients and stir into vegetables.
4. Cook over medium heat, stirring until sauce thickens.

Yield: 4 servings, 2 cups
One Serving = ½ cup

   Calories: 67   Fiber: 1.2 g
   Protein: 2 g   Cholesterol: 0
   Fat: 3 g   Sodium: 192 mg
   Carbohydrate: 8 g   Potassium: 286 mg

Exchange: 2 vegetable
         ½ fat

CAULIFLOWER CURRY

Serve this with rice, spinach pasta, or bread.

1 head cauliflower, coarsely chopped (approximately 3 cups)
1 tablespoon margarine or vegetable oil
4 green onions, chopped
¼ cup all-purpose flour
1½ cups water
½ cup nonfat milk
2 teaspoons curry powder
¼ cup freshly grated low-fat cheese (part-skim mozzarella, Monterey Jack, or Cheddar)

1. Steam cauliflower until tender. Drain and set aside.
2. In large saucepan, melt margarine.
3. Add onion and sauté until soft.
4. Combine flour, water, and milk; stir until well blended, add to onions, and cook until thickened.
5. Add curry and mix well.
6. Stir in cheese and cauliflower.

Yield: 6 servings, 4 cups
One Serving = ⅔ cup

Calories: 71
Protein: 4 g
Fat: 3 g
Carbohydrate: 8 g

Fiber: 2 g
Cholesterol: 3 mg
Sodium: 66 mg
Potassium: 257 mg

Exchange: 1 vegetable
         1 fat

CONFETTI CORN ————————————

1 package (10 ounces) frozen whole kernel corn
6 green onions, chopped, tops included
1 clove garlic, finely chopped
1 teaspoon margarine
1 tablespoon diced pimiento or red pepper

1. Put corn in steamer and place over a pan containing a small amount of water. Cover and cook until tender; drain.
2. Meanwhile, sauté onions and garlic in a saucepan with margarine until tender, about 5 minutes.
3. Add corn and pimiento to onion. Reduce heat and cook 5 minutes longer.

Microwave
1. Cook corn in a microwave oven according to package directions.
2. Add onions, garlic, margarine, and pimiento or red pepper. Cook in microwave on High for 3 minutes.

Yield: 4 servings, 2 cups
One Serving = ½ cup

Calories: 71	Fiber: 5 g*
Protein: 3 g	Cholesterol: 0
Fat: 1 g	Sodium: 16 mg
Carbohydrate: 16 g	Potassium: 159 mg

Exchange: 1 starch/bread

*Good source of dietary fiber

GERMAN POTATO BAKE ────────────────────

4 new potatoes, thinly sliced
Nonstick vegetable spray
¼ cup chopped onions
2 ounces Canadian bacon, diced
1 teaspoon chopped fresh parsley
¼ teaspoon celery seed
1 tablespoon cider vinegar
2 teaspoons margarine
1½ tablespoons all-purpose flour
1½ cups nonfat milk

1. Steam sliced potatoes until slightly tender.
2. Place potatoes in a 10-inch baking dish coated with nonstick vegetable spray and layer with onions, bacon, parsley, celery seed, and vinegar.
3. In a saucepan, melt margarine and add flour, stirring constantly. Cook the flour and margarine for 3 minutes. Do not brown!
4. Stir in milk with a wire whisk and cook slowly until sauce begins to thicken.
5. Pour white sauce over potatoes and bake for 20 to 30 minutes in a 350°F oven, testing tenderness with a fork.

Yield: 8 servings, 4 cups
One Serving = ½ cup

Calories: 104
Protein: 4 g
Fat: 2 g
Carbohydrate: 18 g

Fiber: 1 g
Cholesterol: 5 mg
Sodium: 150 mg
Potassium: 340 mg

Exchange: 1 starch/bread
½ fat

GINGER-LEMON BROCCOLI _____ EASY

1 bunch broccoli (about 1¼ pounds)
1 tablespoon vegetable oil
2 teaspoons minced ginger root
2 tablespoons freshly squeezed lemon juice
Freshly ground black pepper

1. Cut broccoli into ½-inch-thick pieces.
2. Place steamer in a pan containing a small amount of water and steam broccoli for 3 to 5 minutes or until tender.
3. Meanwhile, heat oil in skillet over medium-low heat. Add ginger root and cook for 2 minutes. Stir in lemon juice.
4. Pour lemon-juice mixture over broccoli and sprinkle with pepper to taste.

Yield: 6 servings, about 3 cups
One Serving = ½ cup

Calories: 40	Fiber: 1.5 g
Protein: 2 g	Cholesterol: 0
Fat: 3 g	Sodium: 17 mg
Carbohydrate: 4 g	Potassium: 202 mg

Exchange: 1 vegetable
        ½ fat

GREEN BEANS AND MUSTARD VINAIGRETTE ___ MICROWAVE

1 pound green beans
¼ cup sliced water chestnuts
2 tablespoons chopped onion
2 tablespoons Dijon-style mustard

2 tablespoons vegetable oil
2 tablespoons white vinegar
Salt and freshly ground black
    pepper to taste

1. Place green beans, water chestnuts, and onion in a dish. Cover and cook in the microwave on High for 5 to 7 minutes, or until green beans are tender.
2. In a small, separate dish, heat mustard with oil and vinegar.
3. Pour vinaigrette over vegetables and toss to coat. Serve warm.

Yield: 8 servings, 4 cups
One Serving = ½ cup

Calories: 57
Protein: 1 g
Fat: 4 g
Carbohydrate: 6 g

Fiber: 1 g
Cholesterol: 0
Sodium: 84 mg
Potassium: 187 mg

Exchange: 1 vegetable
½ fat

ITALIAN VEGETABLES

¼ cup chopped onion
1 clove garlic, minced
1 medium zucchini, sliced
1 medium yellow crookneck
squash, sliced
1 green pepper, seeded and sliced

1 teaspoon oregano
1 cup diced mushrooms
1 tomato, cut into wedges
Freshly grated Parmesan cheese
(optional)

1. In large nonstick pan, cook onion and garlic until onion is tender.
2. Stir in zucchini, yellow squash, green pepper, oregano, and mushrooms.
3. Cook, covered, over medium heat, stirring frequently for about 5 minutes or until squash is crisp-tender.
4. Stir in tomato. Cover and cook 1 minute more.
5. Sprinkle with Parmesan cheese if desired. Serve immediately.

Yield: 12 servings, 6 cups
One Serving = ½ cup

Calories: 25
Protein: 2 g
Fat: <1 g
Carbohydrate: 5 g

Fiber: 1.7 g
Cholesterol: 0
Sodium: 6 mg
Potassium: 306 mg

Exchange: 1 vegetable

MARINATED CUCUMBERS ——————————————— EASY

1 medium cucumber, peeled and sliced
½ teaspoon salt
1 small onion, sliced and separated into rings
¼ cup red wine vinegar
1 teaspoon vegetable oil
1 teaspoon dill weed
1 teaspoon minced fresh parsley

Combine all ingredients with 2 tablespoons water. Refrigerate at least 1 hour before serving.

Yield: 4 servings, 2 cups
One Serving = ½ cup

Calories: 26
Protein: <1 g
Fat: 1 g
Carbohydrate: 4 g

Fiber: 1.1 g
Cholesterol: 0
Sodium: 269 mg
Potassium: 134 mg

Exchange: 1 vegetable

MEDITERRANEAN VEGETABLES _____

Marinade
>⅓ **cup olive oil**
>⅓ **cup red wine vinegar**
>¼ **cup finely chopped fresh parsley**
>2 **medium cloves garlic**
>1 **tablespoon Dijon-style mustard**
>1 **teaspoon Equal**
>1 **tablespoon minced fresh basil or** ½ **tablespoon dried**
>¼ **teaspoon salt (optional)**
>⅛ **teaspoon freshly ground black pepper**

>¼ **cup crumbled feta or another skim-milk cheese**
>4 **cups assorted vegetables, such as broccoli, cucumber, snow peas, mushrooms, cherry tomatoes, celery, carrots, asparagus, peppers, green onions, and artichoke hearts**

1. In a blender container, combine all marinade ingredients until smooth.
2. Stir in cheese and pour over vegetables. Toss well.
3. Cover and refrigerate for at least 2 hours.

Yield: 8 servings, 4 cups vegetables, 1 cup marinade
One Serving = ½ cup vegetables with marinade

Calories: 72	Fiber: 1.4 g
Protein: 2 g	Cholesterol: 3 mg
Fat: 6 g	Sodium: 69 mg (without salt)
Carbohydrate: 5 g	Potassium: 191.5 mg

Exchange: 1 vegetable
          1 fat

1 package (10 ounces) frozen chopped spinach
½ cup nonfat or low-fat plain yogurt
2 egg whites
¼ cup freshly grated Parmesan cheese
1 tablespoon finely minced onion
¼ teaspoon oregano
Nonstick vegetable spray

1. Cook spinach according to package directions and drain.
2. Combine next 5 ingredients and pour into a small casserole dish coated with nonstick vegetable spray.
3. Bake at 350°F for 25 to 35 minutes.

Microwave
1. Cook spinach according to microwave instructions on package.
2. Combine next 5 ingredients in a small microwave-safe casserole dish coated with nonstick vegetable spray. Cook in microwave on High for 8 minutes.

Yield: 4 servings, 2 cups
One Serving = ½ cup

Calories: 129
Protein: 14 g
Fat: 4 g
Carbohydrate: 11 g

Fiber: 3.6 g
Cholesterol: 12 mg
Sodium: 361 mg
Potassium: 493 mg

Exchange: 1 vegetable
½ low-fat milk
½ lean meat

RED CABBAGE WITH APPLES

1 tablespoon margarine
2 pounds red cabbage, cored and shredded
1 medium onion, chopped
1½ pounds (about 3 large) tart green apples, cored and chopped
1 teaspoon salt (optional)
2 tablespoons brown sugar
2 tablespoons cider vinegar
¼ teaspoon ground cloves
Pinch of cinnamon
Pinch of nutmeg
Freshly ground black pepper to taste
6 ounces beer

1. Melt margarine in a large saucepan or skillet.
2. Sauté cabbage, onion, and apples in margarine for about 10 minutes, stirring often.
3. Add the salt (if desired), sugar, vinegar, cloves, cinnamon, nutmeg, pepper, and beer.
4. Stir mixture well. Cover and simmer over low heat for 1 hour, stirring occasionally.
5. The cabbage may be served immediately, but for best results, allow to cool for several hours or overnight; then reheat.

Yield: 8 servings, 4 cups
One Serving = ½ cup

Calories: 118
Protein: 1 g
Fat: 2 g
Carbohydrate: 24 g

Fiber: 4.3 g
Cholesterol: 0
Sodium: 279 mg
Potassium: 362 mg

Exchange: 2 vegetable
             1 fruit

STIR-FRIED VEGETABLES _____

¼ cup water
2 teaspoons cornstarch
2 tablespoons soy sauce
¼ teaspoon ginger
¼ teaspoon nutmeg
1 tablespoon olive oil
½ medium onion, sliced and separated into rings
1 cup finely chopped bok choy (Chinese cabbage)
1 clove garlic, pressed
1 cup chopped mushrooms
1 can (8 ounces) bamboo shoots, drained
1 can (8¾ ounces) baby sweet corn, drained
1 can (8 ounces) water chestnuts, drained
1 cup chopped broccoli
1 cup chopped red pepper or pimiento

1. In a small bowl, mix the first 5 ingredients together and set aside.
2. Heat large skillet or wok over high heat; add olive oil.
3. Stir-fry onion rings, bok choy, and garlic in hot oil for 1 to 2 minutes. Remove the mixture from wok or skillet. Set aside.
4. Place mushrooms, bamboo shoots, baby corn, and water chestnuts in the wok or skillet. Stir-fry for about 2 minutes.
5. Add the soy mixture and cook until bubbly, stirring frequently. Add broccoli and red pepper, cover, and cook for 3 minutes or until broccoli is crisp-tender. Stir in onion, bok choy, and garlic and serve.

Yield: 6 servings, 6 cups
One Serving = 1 cup

Calories: 104	Fiber: 4 g
Protein: 4 g	Cholesterol: 0
Fat: 3 g	Sodium: 497 mg*
Carbohydrate: 19 g	Potassium: 350 mg

Exchange: ½ starch/bread
            2 vegetable

*High in sodium

STUFFED ACORN SQUASH ⎯⎯⎯⎯⎯⎯⎯ MICROWAVE

Makes a great meatless lunch or dinner entree if you double the portion size.

> **1 large red onion, chopped**
> **1 cup cooked brown rice**
> **¾ cup freshly grated part-skim mozzarella cheese**
> **¼ teaspoon salt**
> **½ teaspoon freshly ground black pepper**
> **2 tablespoons minced fresh parsley**
> **2 acorn squash, halved and seeded**

1. Combine first 6 ingredients in a large bowl and set aside.
2. Place squash, cut side down, in a microwave-safe baking dish. Cover with lid or plastic wrap and cook for 8 minutes on high.
3. Remove dish and turn squash cut side up. Fill squash halves with rice mixture. Cover and cook an additional 6 to 8 minutes on high, or until heated thoroughly.
4. Remove cover and let stand for 5 minutes to finish cooking.

Yield: 4 servings
One Serving = ½ squash

Calories: 203	Fiber: 7 g*
Protein: 9 g	Cholesterol: 11 mg
Fat: 5 g	Sodium: 249 mg
Carbohydrate: 32 g	Potassium: 429 mg

Exchange: 1 starch/bread
1 medium-fat meat
2 vegetable

*Good source of dietary fiber

STUFFED GREEN PEPPERS _____

⅓ cup long-grain rice
⅔ cup water
4 green peppers, stemmed and seeded
1½ cups spaghetti sauce (low-sodium)
¼ teaspoon garlic powder
¼ teaspoon onion powder
1 tablespoon freshly grated Parmesan cheese

1. Combine rice and water in a saucepan and bring to a boil. Reduce heat to simmer, cover, and cook for about 15 minutes.
2. Steam green peppers, or cook in microwave, until tender.
3. Combine rice with 1 cup of the spaghetti sauce, and the garlic and onion powders.
4. Fill green peppers with rice mixture; place in a baking dish.
5. Pour the remaining ½ cup of spaghetti sauce over the peppers.
6. Sprinkle with Parmesan cheese.
7. Place in a preheated 325°F oven for about 20 minutes or until heated thoroughly.

Yield: 4 servings, 4 peppers
One Serving = 1 pepper

Calories: 135	Fiber: 3.4 g
Protein: 3 g	Cholesterol: 1 mg
Fat: 4 g	Sodium: 48 mg
Carbohydrate: 23 g	Potassium: 578 mg

Exchange: ½ starch/bread
2 vegetable
1 fat

STUFFED TOMATOES ——————————————————— QUICK

   4 medium tomatoes
   2 green onions, chopped
   1 cup water chestnuts
   2 tablespoons whole wheat bread crumbs, Italian style
   2 tablespoons freshly grated Parmesan cheese
   3 tablespoons reduced-calorie mayonnaise
   2 teaspoons oregano
   2 tablespoons chopped fresh parsley

1. Cut tops off tomatoes, scoop out centers (save for other uses).
Turn shells upside down to drain.
2. Combine the remaining ingredients, except parsley, in a bowl. Mix
well.
3. Fill each tomato shell with ¼ cup of the mixture.
4. Sprinkle each shell with parsley.
5. Broil 5 minutes until heated through.

Yield: 4 servings, 4 tomatoes, 1 cup mixture
One Serving = 1 tomato with ¼ cup mixture

   Calories: 113   Fiber: 4.1 g
   Protein: 4 g   Cholesterol: 6 mg
   Fat: 5 g   Sodium: 156 mg
   Carbohydrate: 17 g   Potassium: 484 mg

Exchange: 2 vegetable
         1 fat

ZUCCHINI BOATS _____ MICROWAVE

Serve as an accompaniment to your favorite pasta dish or increase the portion size for a meatless entree.

1 large zucchini (about 8 inches)
1 tablespoon chopped mushrooms
1 tablespoon chopped onion
2 tablespoons chopped green pepper
½ tomato, diced
½ clove garlic, finely minced
1 teaspoon oregano
2 teaspoons freshly grated Parmesan cheese

1. Slice zucchini in half lengthwise.
2. Scoop out center, leaving a ¼-inch-thick "boat." Dice the zucchini from the center.
3. Toss together mushrooms, onion, pepper, tomato, garlic, oregano, and diced zucchini.
4. Fill zucchini boats with vegetable mixture.
5. Place boats in a microwave-safe baking dish. Add 2 tablespoons water to the bottom.
6. Sprinkle with Parmesan cheese.
7. Cover dish with plastic wrap. Cook on High for 10 to 12 minutes or until boats are tender when pierced with a fork.
8. Remove and let stand for 5 minutes to finish cooking.

Yield: 2 medium boats
One Serving = 1 medium boat

Calories: 43	Fiber: 2.6 g
Protein: 3 g	Cholesterol: 1.3 mg
Fat: <1 g	Sodium: 39 mg
Carbohydrate: 8 g	Potassium: 510 mg

Exchange: 2 vegetable

12

BREADS

This section offers a wide variety of bread choices, including muffins, quick breads, pretzels, crêpes, tortillas, and crackers. We have tried to maximize the use of whole grains and whole grain flours in our recipes to increase their nutritional value and fiber content. Some feature grains that are relatively new on the market — oat bran, blue cornmeal, and amaranth flour.

There is very little that compares with freshly baked bread! Try our recipes with little or no margarine and appreciate their true flavor.

Apple Date Nut Bread
Banamaranth Muffins
Bean Bread
Bran Brown Bread
Bread Sticks
Buttermilk Scones
Crescent Roll Snacks
Crunchy Wheat Bread
French Toast Bake
Garlic Cheese Casserole
   Bread

Oat Bran Crackers
Old-Fashioned Wheat Pretzels
Parmesan Herb Bread
Popovers
Pumpkin Rolls
Whole Wheat Pan Bread
Santa Fe Blue Cornmeal
   Bread
Whole Wheat Tortillas

APPLE DATE NUT BREAD _____

This high-fiber yeast bread is easy to assemble since it does not require kneading. Loaves keep well when covered with plastic wrap.
Freeze those you will not eat within the next two or three days.

2 tablespoons active dry yeast	**1 tablespoon cinnamon**
¼ cup warm water (110°F)	**1 teaspoon allspice**
⅓ cup vegetable oil	**1 teaspoon nutmeg**
2 eggs or egg equivalent	**½ cup fructose**
1 cup unsweetened applesauce	**¼ cup nonfat milk**
1½ cups whole wheat flour	**⅓ cup pitted and chopped dates**
1½ cups unbleached all-purpose	**⅓ cup coarsely chopped walnuts**
flour	**(optional)**
1 cup instant oats	**Nonstick vegetable spray**

1. Dissolve yeast in warm water. Let stand until yeast bubbles.
2. In a separate bowl combine oil, eggs, and applesauce. Add yeast
mixture.
3. In a large bowl, mix together flours, oats, spices, and fructose.
4. Gradually stir flour mixture into wet ingredients. Combine well.
Add nonfat milk to moisten dough.
5. Stir in dates and walnuts (if desired).
6. Pour into 2 standard loaf pans or 3 small loaf pans coated with
nonstick vegetable spray.
7. Cover with a towel and place in a warm, draft-free area to rise, 45
minutes to 1 hour.
8. Bake in a preheated 350°F oven for 45 minutes or until loaves are
golden brown and a knife inserted in center of loaf comes out clean.

Yield: 2 loaves, 10 slices per loaf
One Serving = 1 slice, ¹⁄₁₀ of loaf (without nuts)

Calories: 163	Fiber: 2.2 g
Protein: 4 g	Cholesterol: 29 mg
Fat: 5 g	Sodium: 52 mg
Carbohydrate: 27 g	Potassium: 120 mg

Exchange: 1½ starch/bread
            1 fat

BANAMARANTH MUFFINS ────────────

An exciting new recipe using high-protein, high-fiber amaranth flour. The Aztecs discovered this nutritious grain centuries ago. Rich in calcium, iron, and phosphorus, it combines well with other flours in your favorite baked recipes.

Nonstick vegetable spray	3 tablespoons brown sugar
1 cup whole wheat flour	1 egg
½ cup amaranth flour	2 small ripe bananas, mashed
2 teaspoons baking powder	(about 1 cup)
¼ teaspoon baking soda	¼ cup apple juice
½ teaspoon cinnamon	1 tablespoon finely chopped
3 tablespoons vegetable margarine	walnuts

1. Preheat oven to 400°F. Spray a 12-cup muffin tin with nonstick vegetable spray.
2. Combine the flours, baking powder, baking soda, and cinnamon in a bowl.
3. Beat together the margarine and sugar until light and fluffy. Beat in the egg.
4. Mix in the dry ingredients and alternate with the mashed bananas and apple juice. Stir in the nuts.
5. Spoon the batter into the muffin cups, filling two thirds full.
6. Bake for 20 minutes or until golden brown. Remove to a wire rack for cooling.

Yield: 12 muffins
One Serving = 1 muffin

Calories: 148	Fiber: 1 g
Protein: 3 g	Cholesterol: 23 mg
Fat: 5 g	Sodium: 81 mg
Carbohydrate: 24 g	Potassium: 118 mg

Exchange: 1½ starch/bread
        1 fat

BEAN BREAD

The addition of beans makes this a high-protein bread loaded with fiber. Add your favorite legume to create your own unique variation.

1 package active dry yeast
2 tablespoons honey
½ cup warm water (110°F)
⅛ cup vegetable oil
1 cup cooked or canned and mashed lentils, kidney or pinto beans

1½ cups unbleached all-purpose flour
1 cup whole wheat flour
1 teaspoon salt
Nonstick vegetable spray

1. Combine yeast, honey, and warm water in a bowl. Let set until bubbly.
2. Combine the yeast mixture with the oil and beans in a large bowl.
3. Gradually stir in the flours and salt.
4. Add additional water (2 to 4 tablespoons) if the dough is too dry.
5. Turn the dough onto a floured board and knead for 10 minutes or until smooth and elastic. Place in a lightly oiled bowl. Cover with a towel and let rise in a warm area until doubled in size (about 1 hour).
6. Punch down dough, knead briefly, and let rise a second time until doubled in size (about 45 minutes).
7. Form into a loaf shape and place in a greased 9 × 5-inch loaf pan coated with nonstick vegetable spray.
8. Bake in a preheated 350°F oven for 50 to 60 minutes or until the crust is golden brown.
9. Remove from the pan and let cool on a rack.

Yield: 1 loaf, 15 slices
One Serving = 1 slice

Calories: 110
Protein: 4 g
Fat: 2 g
Carbohydrate: 20 g

Fiber: 1.9 g
Cholesterol: 0
Sodium: 143 mg
Potassium: 99 mg

Exchange: 1½ starch/bread

BRAN BROWN BREAD

This bread has a rich, spicy taste. It goes well with a thin layer of Creamy Cheese Spread on top (p. 322).

⅓ cup margarine
3 tablespoons apple juice
2 egg whites
1 cup unbleached all-purpose flour
¾ cup whole wheat flour
1½ teaspoons baking soda
½ teaspoon baking powder

½ teaspoon salt
⅛ teaspoon cinnamon
1 cup less 2 tablespoons water
3 tablespoons dark molasses
½ cup raisins
1 cup wheat bran flakes
1 teaspoon vanilla
Nonstick vegetable spray

1. Mix margarine, apple juice, and egg whites together until well blended.
2. Sift together the flours, soda, baking powder, salt, and cinnamon in a separate bowl.
3. Add the flour mixture to the apple juice mixture alternately with the water and molasses.
4. Add raisins, wheat bran flakes, and vanilla. Combine until batter is thoroughly moistened. Do not overmix.
5. Pour into a 9 × 5-inch loaf pan coated with nonstick spray and bake in a preheated 350°F oven for 1 hour.

Yield: 1 loaf, 12 slices
One Serving = 1 slice

Calories: 147
Protein: 3 g
Fat: 5 g
Carbohydrate: 23 g

Fiber: 1.9 g
Cholesterol: 0
Sodium: 310 mg
Potassium: 266 mg

Exchange: 1 starch/bread
½ fruit
1 fat

BREAD STICKS

Vary the length of these bread sticks: when long they make a dramatic accompaniment to a simple pasta meal; when short they become the perfect appetizer with your favorite dip.

3 to 3½ cups all-purpose flour
1 tablespoon sugar
1 teaspoon salt
2 packages active dry yeast
1¼ cups warm water (110°F)

¼ cup olive oil
Nonstick vegetable spray
1 egg white beaten with 1
   tablespoon water
Toasted sesame or poppy seeds
   (optional)

1. In a large bowl, stir together 1 cup of the flour, sugar, salt, and yeast. Gradually add warm water, oil, and beat at medium speed with an electric mixer for 2 minutes.
2. Add ½ cup more flour and beat at high speed for 2 minutes. Stir in 1½ to 2 cups of remaining flour to make a soft dough.
3. On a floured board, with floured hands, shape dough into a ball and divide into 16 to 20 equal pieces for long bread sticks or 40 equal pieces for appetizer bread sticks. Roll each piece into a 12-inch, 16-inch, or 20-inch rope. Place on a baking sheet that you have coated with nonstick spray.
4. Set bread sticks in a warm place, cover with a towel, and let rise until puffy, about 15 minutes. Brush each stick gently with egg-water mixture; then sprinkle with sesame or poppy seeds, if desired.
5. Bake in a preheated 375°F oven for 15 to 20 minutes or until lightly browned.

Yield: 40 12-inch sticks or 16 to 20 18-inch sticks
One Serving = 1 12-inch stick

Calories: 64
Protein: 2 g
Fat: 2 g
Carbohydrate: 11 g

Fiber: 0.7 g
Cholesterol: 0
Sodium: 55 mg
Potassium: 23 mg

Exchange: 1 starch/bread

NOTE: You can freeze these bread sticks easily and bake them at a later date. After you shape the sticks, cover them tightly with plastic wrap and seal into plastic freezer storage bags. Store in freezer up to 4 weeks. Remove frozen sticks from freezer and let thaw for 30 minutes. Place on an ungreased baking sheet and let thaw fully, about 15 minutes. Bake as above.

BUTTERMILK SCONES

Serve these scones at breakfast, brunch, or tea time with dietetic jelly or apple butter and an assortment of fresh fruits.

1½ cups all-purpose flour
1½ cups old-fashioned oats or 1¼ cups quick oats
3 tablespoons sugar
1 tablespoon baking powder
1 teaspoon cream of tartar
½ teaspoon salt
⅓ cup unsalted safflower margarine, melted
⅔ cup low-fat buttermilk
1 egg
½ cup raisins or currants
Nonstick vegetable spray

1. Preheat oven to 425°F.
2. Combine first 6 ingredients. Add margarine, buttermilk, and egg. Mix just until the dry ingredients are moistened.
3. Stir in the raisins.
4. With your hands, shape the dough to form a ball. Pat out on a lightly floured surface to form an 8-inch circle. Cut into 12 wedges.
5. Bake on a cookie sheet coated with nonstick vegetable spray for 12 to 15 minutes or until light brown.
6. Serve warm.

Yield: 12 scones
One Serving = 1 scone

Calories: 179
Protein: 4 g
Fat: 7 g
Carbohydrate: 26 g

Fiber: 1.5 g
Cholesterol: 24 mg
Sodium: 202 mg
Potassium: 137 mg

Exchange: 1½ starch/bread
          1 fat

CRESCENT ROLL SNACKS _____

These crunchy little breads are delicious as between-meal nibbles or with a main meal, soup, or salad.

2 packages active dry yeast	3 cups unbleached all-purpose
3 tablespoons honey	flour, wheat flour, or a
1 cup warm water (110°F)	combination of both
5 ounces evaporated skim milk	Nonstick vegetable spray
1 teaspoon salt (optional)	1 egg white, lightly beaten
2 teaspoons vegetable oil	2 tablespoons caraway seeds

1. In a large bowl, dissolve yeast and honey in warm water. Let sit 5 to 10 minutes until bubbly. Add milk, salt (if desired), and oil. Mix well.

2. Gradually stir in 3 cups flour until a soft dough is formed. Turn dough out onto a lightly floured surface and knead until smooth (about 10 minutes).

3. Place dough into a bowl coated with nonstick vegetable spray; cover and let rise until doubled (about 1 hour).

4. Punch dough down, knead for 1 to 2 minutes, then divide dough into 4 equal parts. Cover and let rest for 10 minutes.

5. Roll each part into a 10-inch circle and cut with a knife into 8 wedges. Starting at wide end, roll each wedge into a crescent shape and place onto a baking sheet coated with nonstick spray.

6. Brush tops with egg white and sprinkle with caraway seeds. Let rise for 30 minutes or until crescents are puffy.

7. Bake in a preheated 400°F oven for 15 minutes or until crusts are golden.

Yield: 32 crescents
One Serving = 1 crescent

Calories: 61	Fiber: 0
Protein: 2 g	Cholesterol: 0
Fat: <1 g	Sodium: 68 mg
Carbohydrate: 12 g	Potassium: 47 mg

Exchange: 1 starch/bread

CRUNCHY WHEAT BREAD

A good basic yeast bread. Be creative and mix other types of flours and grains to give the bread a different flavor.

1 package active dry yeast	3 tablespoons margarine
1½ cups warm water (110°F)	½ cup rye flour or ½ cup whole
5½ to 6 cups whole wheat flour	wheat graham flour or ¼ cup
¼ cup honey	wheat germ + ¼ cup wheat
½ cup hot water	bran
2 teaspoons salt (optional)	Nonstick vegetable spray

1. Dissolve the yeast in the warm water. Add 2 cups of the whole wheat flour and 2 tablespoons of the honey. Stir and set aside in a warm place for 20 minutes.

2. Combine the hot water, salt (if desired), margarine, and the remainder of the honey. Mix and let cool. Add to the yeast mixture.

3. Stir in rye flour or other variation. Add the remaining whole wheat flour, ½ cup at a time, until the dough is ready for kneading.

4. Knead dough on a lightly floured surface for about 10 minutes or until dough is elastic. Place dough in a bowl coated with nonstick spray. Cover with a towel and place in a warm, draft-free area for about 1½ hours or until doubled in size.

5. Punch dough down and knead for 2 minutes on a floured surface. Shape dough into 2 loaves and place in loaf pans coated with nonstick spray. Cover and let rise until doubled in size, about 45 minutes.

6. Bake in a preheated 350°F oven for 35 minutes or until tops are golden brown. Cool on wire racks.

Yield: 2 medium-size loaves; 10 slices per loaf
One Serving = 1 slice

Calories: 157	Fiber: 3.5 g
Protein: 5 g	Cholesterol: 0
Fat: 2 g	Sodium: 235 mg
Carbohydrate: 31 g	Potassium: 148 mg

Exchange: 2 starch/bread

FRENCH TOAST BAKE

A quick idea for brunch. It can bake while you prepare the Fruit Syrup (p. 291). Serve with unsweetened applesauce or dietetic syrup.

2 eggs, beaten
⅓ cup nonfat milk
1 teaspoon vanilla
1 teaspoon sugar
⅛ teaspoon cinnamon
10 slices French bread, cut into ¾-inch-thick rounds

1. In a shallow dish, combine eggs, milk, vanilla, sugar, and cinnamon.
2. Dip bread slices into milk mixture, coating both sides. Allow excess to drain.
3. Place slices on a nonstick baking sheet.
4. Bake in a preheated 400°F oven for 10 minutes on each side or until golden brown.

Yield: 10 baguette slices
One Serving = 2 slices

Calories: 110	Fiber: 0
Protein: 5 g	Cholesterol: 110 mg
Fat: 3 g	Sodium: 174 mg
Carbohydrate: 14 g	Potassium: 76 mg

Exchange: 1 starch/bread
         ½ fat

GARLIC CHEESE CASSEROLE BREAD ⎯⎯⎯⎯⎯⎯⎯⎯⎯⎯

A delicious "no-knead" yeast bread. The addition of cottage cheese gives this bread a moist texture.

1 package active dry yeast	1 tablespoon oregano
½ cup warm water (110°F)	2 teaspoons honey
1 cup low-fat cottage cheese	1 teaspoon salt (optional)
4 cloves garlic, minced	¼ teaspoon baking soda
1 egg	2½ cups flour
1 tablespoon olive oil	Nonstick vegetable spray

1. Dissolve the yeast in the water.

2. In a saucepan over medium temperature, heat the cottage cheese until warm.

3. Pour the heated cottage cheese into a large mixing bowl and combine with yeast, garlic, egg, oil, oregano, honey, salt (if desired), and baking soda.

4. Add the flour and blend well with wooden spoon or in a food processor. Batter will be sticky.

5. Transfer the batter into a large bowl coated with nonstick spray; cover with a towel and let rise in a warm, draft-free area for about 1 hour.

6. Stir with a spoon and turn into a 2-quart casserole dish coated with nonstick spray. Let rise for 30 minutes.

7. Bake in a preheated 350°F oven for 40 minutes or until done.

8. To serve, remove to a platter or spoon out of the casserole dish.

Yield: 1 loaf, 20 squares
One Serving = 1 square

Calories: 77	Fiber: 0.7 g
Protein: 4 g	Cholesterol: 15 mg
Fat: 1 g	Sodium: 167 mg
Carbohydrate: 12 g	Potassium: 41 mg

Exchange: 1 starch/bread

OAT BRAN CRACKERS

A low-fat alternative to commercial crackers. Another added benefit is the high fiber content of the oat bran.

½ cup old-fashioned oats
½ cup oat bran
½ cup whole wheat flour
½ teaspoon salt
⅛ teaspoon baking soda

1 tablespoon margarine, melted
1 teaspoon honey
½ cup boiling water
Nonstick vegetable spray

1. Grind rolled oats in a food processor or blender until fine.
2. Combine ground oats with other dry ingredients in a bowl. Add melted margarine, honey, and water, and stir with a fork until well mixed.
3. Form dough into a ball with your hands; press firmly.
4. On a floured board, roll out dough until thin. Cut dough into 2½- to 3-inch circles.
5. Place crackers on a baking sheet coated with nonstick vegetable spray.
6. Bake crackers in a preheated 350°F oven until light brown, about 15 to 20 minutes.
7. Cool on a rack; store in an airtight container.

Yield: 24 crackers
One Serving = 3 crackers

Calories: 77
Protein: 3 g
Fat: 2 g
Carbohydrate: 12 g

Fiber: 1.7 g
Cholesterol: 0
Sodium: 164 mg
Potassium: 78 mg

Exchange: 1 starch/bread

OLD-FASHIONED WHEAT PRETZELS —————————————

Take these pretzels to your next baseball game or tailgate party.
Serve with prepared mustard.

1 package active dry yeast
1 teaspoon honey
½ teaspoon salt (optional)
1½ cups warm water (110°F)
2½ cups unbleached all-purpose
**   flour**

1½ cups whole wheat flour
Nonstick vegetable spray
1 egg white, lightly beaten
1 tablespoon cold water

1. Dissolve yeast, honey, and salt (if desired) in warm water. Beat in
all-purpose flour, stirring for 3 minutes. Add whole wheat flour until
a soft dough is formed.
2. Turn dough onto a floured surface and knead until elastic and
smooth, about 5 minutes. Place in a bowl coated with nonstick vegetable spray, cover with a cloth, and place in a warm, draft-free area
for 1 hour or until doubled in size.
3. Punch dough down. Divide dough in half, then separate each half
into 6 equal portions. Roll each portion into a rope about 15 inches
long.
4. Place each rope onto a baking sheet lightly coated with nonstick
vegetable spray and form a pretzel by bringing the left end of the rope
over its middle, making a loop. Bring the right end of the rope up and
over the first loop. Be sure that the holes between the loops are large
enough so that they do not bake together.
5. Brush tops of pretzels with a mixture of beaten egg white and cold
water.
6. Bake in a preheated 425°F oven for 15 to 20 minutes. Place on a
wire rack and let cool.

Yield: 12 pretzels
One Serving = 1 pretzel

Calories: 143
Protein: 5 g
Fat: 1 g
Carbohydrate: 29 g

Fiber: 1.9 g
Cholesterol: 23 mg
Sodium: 88 mg
Potassium: 100 mg

Exchange: 2 starch/bread

PARMESAN HERB BREAD

Try substituting other fresh herbs like dill, basil, or rosemary.

2½ cups all-purpose flour
¾ teaspoon salt, or less
½ teaspoon baking soda
2 teaspoons baking powder
⅛ teaspoon cayenne pepper
(optional)
1 teaspoon sage or poultry
seasoning
1 teaspoon coarsely ground black
pepper

1 cup freshly grated Parmesan
cheese
¾ cup minced fresh parsley
3 tablespoons margarine, softened
2 tablespoons sugar
4 egg whites or 2 egg equivalents
1¼ cup buttermilk
½ teaspoon Worcestershire sauce
Nonstick vegetable spray

1. In a bowl, combine the flour, salt, baking soda, baking powder, cayenne (if desired), sage, black pepper, Parmesan, and parsley.
2. In a separate bowl, stir together the margarine, sugar, and egg whites. Add the buttermilk and the Worcestershire sauce and combine thoroughly.
3. Add the flour mixture to the liquids and stir the batter until it is just moistened.
4. Pour batter into a 9 × 5 × 3-inch loaf pan, or a 12-cup muffin tin, coated with nonstick spray.
5. Bake in a preheated 350°F oven for 40 to 45 minutes or until done. Let the loaf cool in the pan for 10 minutes.

Yield: 1 loaf (12 slices) or 12 muffins
One Serving = 1 slice or 1 muffin

Calories: 174
Protein: 7 g
Fat: 6 g
Carbohydrate: 22 g

Fiber: 1 g
Cholesterol: 9 mg
Sodium: 386 mg (with ¾
teaspoon salt)
Potassium: 110 mg

Exchange: 1½ starch/bread
1 fat

POPOVERS _____

These popovers taste best piping hot from the oven. Serve at tea time with apple butter. For a light breakfast treat, spread with part-skim ricotta cheese.

> ½ **cup sifted all-purpose flour**
> ½ **cup sifted whole wheat flour**
> ¼ **teaspoon salt (optional)**
> **1 egg**
> **4 egg whites**
> **1 cup low-fat milk**
> **1 tablespoon margarine, melted**
> **Nonstick vegetable spray**

1. Preheat oven to 425°F.
2. Combine flours, salt (if desired), egg, egg whites, milk, and melted margarine. Mix for about 2½ minutes, until very smooth.
3. Coat 6 muffin cups or popover pans with nonstick vegetable spray and fill each cup half full with the batter.
4. Bake for 20 minutes. Do not open the oven door at this point, or the popovers will collapse.
5. Reduce the temperature to 325°F and bake an additional 20 minutes, or until crust is golden brown.
6. Remove the popovers from the tins and serve immediately.

Yield: 6 popovers
One Serving = 1 popover

Calories: 129	Fiber: 1.2 g
Protein: 7 g	Cholesterol: 49 mg
Fat: 4 g	Sodium: 177 mg
Carbohydrate: 17 g	Potassium: 151 mg

Exchange: 1 starch/bread
           1 fat

PUMPKIN ROLLS

A great holiday favorite.

1 package active dry yeast
1 cup warm water (110°F)
⅓ cup honey
2 tablespoons margarine
1 teaspoon salt
½ cup nonfat dry milk
1 cup canned pumpkin
1½ teaspoons cinnamon

¾ teaspoon ground cloves
¾ teaspoon nutmeg
¾ teaspoon ginger
2½ to 3 cups unbleached all-purpose flour
1½ to 2 cups whole wheat flour
Nonstick vegetable spray

1. In a large bowl or food processor, dissolve yeast in water. Add honey, margarine, salt, dry milk, pumpkin, cinnamon, cloves, nutmeg, and ginger. Beat well to blend, then gradually beat in about 4 cups of the combined flours to make a stiff dough.
2. Turn dough out onto a floured board and knead until smooth (about 15 to 20 minutes), adding flour as needed to prevent sticking.
3. Turn dough over in a bowl coated with nonstick spray, cover, and let rise in a warm place until doubled (approximately 1½ to 2 hours). Punch down dough; knead briefly on a lightly floured board to release air.
4. Divide dough into 24 equal pieces. Shape each into a smooth ball and place balls in 2 greased 9-inch round baking pans coated with nonstick spray. Cover and let rise until almost double.
5. Bake in a preheated 375°F oven for 25 minutes or until browned. Cool on racks.

Yield: 24 rolls
One Serving = 1 roll

Calories: 121
Protein: 3 g
Fat: 1 g
Carbohydrate: 24 g

Fiber: 0.3 g
Cholesterol: 0
Sodium: 103 mg
Potassium: 82 mg

Exchange: 1½ starch/bread

WHOLE WHEAT PAN BREAD

Here is a delicious wheat bread to try when you do not have time to bake a yeast bread.

1½ cups whole wheat flour
1 cup unbleached all-purpose flour
½ cup old-fashioned or quick oats
3 tablespoons brown sugar
1 tablespoon grated orange peel
2 teaspoons baking powder
½ teaspoon baking soda
1¾ cups nonfat milk
1 egg white
¼ cup + 1 tablespoon chopped walnuts
1 teaspoon honey
Poppy or sesame seeds (optional)

1. Preheat oven to 350°F. In a large bowl combine flours, oats, brown sugar, orange peel, baking powder, and baking soda until well blended. Add milk and egg white, stirring only until ingredients are moistened. Fold in ¼ cup of the walnuts.
2. Lightly oil a 1½-quart round casserole dish; sprinkle with the remaining 1 tablespoon of walnuts. Pour batter into prepared dish.
3. Bake for 45 to 60 minutes or until a knife inserted in the center of the bread comes out clean. If necessary, cover loaf with foil during the last 15 minutes of baking to prevent overbrowning.
4. Cool in casserole dish for 10 minutes; turn bread out onto a wire rack. Brush top of loaf with honey and sprinkle with poppy or sesame seeds, if desired. Serve warm or at room temperature.

Yield: 1 loaf, 14 slices
One Serving = 1 slice

Calories: 150
Protein: 5 g
Fat: 4 g
Carbohydrate: 24 g

Fiber: 2 g
Cholesterol: 0.6 mg
Sodium: 93 mg
Potassium: 165 mg

Exchange: 1½ starch/bread
　　　　　 1 fat

SANTA FE BLUE CORNMEAL BREAD ———————————

You can purchase blue cornmeal in most health food stores. This bread makes a nice accompaniment to soup or salad.

¼ cup margarine	1 tablespoon baking powder
1 tablespoon fructose or honey	½ teaspoon salt (optional)
2 egg whites	½ cup nonfat milk
1 egg	¼ cup water
1 cup all-purpose flour	Nonstick vegetable spray
½ cup blue cornmeal	

1. Cream together margarine and fructose.
2. Add egg whites and egg and beat well.
3. Sift together flour, cornmeal, baking powder, and salt (if desired).
4. Combine milk and water.
5. Add half of the dry ingredients and half of the liquid mixture to the egg mixture and beat well. Add remaining dry ingredients and liquid mixture and beat until blended.
6. Spread batter in an 8-inch-square baking pan coated with nonstick spray. Bake in a preheated 400°F oven for 20 to 25 minutes.

Yield: 8 servings
One Serving = 1 square

Calories: 163	Fiber: 1.1 g
Protein: 4 g	Cholesterol: 35 mg
Fat: 7 g	Sodium: 338 mg
Carbohydrate: 21 g	Potassium: 74 mg

Exchange: 1½ starch/bread
          1 fat

WHOLE WHEAT TORTILLAS

These tortillas are lower in saturated fat, with no cholesterol, and higher in fiber than traditional tortillas prepared with lard and white flour.

1½ cups unbleached all-purpose flour
1½ cups whole wheat flour
¼ teaspoon baking powder
1 cup warm water (110°F)
2 teaspoons vegetable oil
¼ teaspoon salt
Cornstarch for dusting the tortillas

1. Stir together the first 6 ingredients.
2. On a floured board, knead until smooth.
3. Divide dough into 12 equal balls. Dust lightly with cornstarch.
4. Roll into a circle as thin as possible on a lightly floured board.
5. Drop onto a very hot ungreased griddle. Cook until brown spots appear on one side.
6. Turn and cook on second side.

Yield: 12 large tortillas
One Serving = 1 tortilla

Calories: 133	Fiber: 1.8 g
Protein: 4 g	Cholesterol: 0
Fat: 1 g	Sodium: 51 mg
Carbohydrate: 27 g	Potassium: 69 mg

Exchange: 1½ starch/bread

13

GRAINS, BEANS, AND PASTA

THE FOODS in this section are staples for much of the world's population. They are a valuable addition to anyone's diet because of their vitamin, mineral, and fiber content (both soluble and insoluble). Grains, beans, and pasta are a natural substitute as Americans learn to moderate their meat, fish, and poultry intake.

Our recipes will provide you with a variety of new ideas on how to incorporate more grains, beans, and pastas into your diet. Feel free to improvise and modify a recipe to incorporate your favorites. Tables 19 and 20 will help you shop for and cook quite a range of grains and beans.

Angel Hair Sauté
Black Beans
Cheesy Broccoli and Pasta
Chili Rice
Bulgur Pilaf
Frijoles de la Olla (Boiled
    Mexican Beans)
Frijoles Refritos (Refried
    Beans)

Insalata Pasta Fredda (Cold
    Pasta Salad)
Meatless White Bean Bake
Muesli
Peppery Pasta
Red Beans and Rice
Spanish Rice

Table 19 Grain Guidelines

Grains	Water (per 1 cup dry)	Cooking Time	Approximate Yield	Part Two Recipe	Comments
Amaranth	3 c	25 min	2½ c	Banamaranth Muffins	Ancient grain of Aztecs. High in protein, fiber, vitamins, and minerals; combines well with other flours in baked goods.
Barley (whole)	3 c	1¼ hr	3½ c	Hearty Lamb and Barley Stew	One of the first domestic grains with a variety of uses; good alone or in soups and casseroles.
Brown Rice	2 c	1 hr	3 c	Spanish Rice, Chili Rice	Versatile grain and staple of many countries; higher in fiber and protein than white rice; good as an accompaniment to main dishes.
Bulgur Wheat (cracked wheat)	2 c	15–20 min	2½ c	Easy Bulgur Pilaf, Tabbouli	Parboiled wheat that has been cracked, it is found in specialty and health food stores; nutty flavor; good as a side dish or in soups, salads, or casseroles.
Cornmeal (coarse)	4 c	25 min	3 c	Polenta Appetizer Squares, Santa Fe Blue Cornmeal Bread	Popular in Mexican cuisine as basis for tortilla; good in muffins and bread.
Oats (flaked, rolled, oatmeal)	3 c	30 min	2½ c	Muesli, Apple Oatmeal Muffins	Popular grain used in cereals and baked products; high in soluble fiber linked to lowering blood cholesterol levels.
Wild Rice	3 c	1 hr or more	4 c	California Wild Rice	Rich in fiber, protein, B vitamins and minerals; an alternative to brown or white rice.

Table 20 Bean Basics

Bean	Description	Water (per 1 cup dry)	Cooking Time	Approximate Yield	Part Two Recipe	Comments
Black	Small, round, earthy flavor	4 c	1½ hr	2 c	Black Beans	Used in South American, Mediterranean, and Chinese dishes; makes good sauces and soups.
Garbanzo (chickpea)	Medium, round, nutty tasting, crunchy, firm texture	4 c	3 hr	2 c	Falafel	Popular in Middle Eastern dishes like hummus; texture holds up well to cooking; good in salads.
Kidney	Red, smooth, kidney-shaped, soft texture	3 c	1½ hr	2 c	Beef and Bean Chili, Fiesta Bean Salad, Red Beans and Rice	Bean most often used in chili; use interchangeably with pinto bean; try in salads and soups.
Lentil	Small, round, smooth, green-brown or red, distinctive taste	3 c	1 hr	2¼ c	Lentil Soup, Spicy Lentils	Quick to prepare — no pre-soaking needed; good in soups or curries.

Bean	Description	Water (per 1 cup dry)	Cooking Time	Approximate Yield	Part Two Recipe	Comments
Peas (split, whole)	Small, oval, soft, yellow or green, distinctive taste	3 c	45 min	2½ c	Split Pea Soup	Excellent in hearty soups and casseroles.
Pinto	Smooth, oval, brown with dark specks, mild taste and texture	3 c	2½ hr	2 c	Pinto Bean Cake, Frijoles de la Olla, Frijoles Refritos	Bean most often used in Mexican dishes; use interchangeably with kidney bean.
Soybeans	Round, nutty taste, firm texture	3 c	3 hr	2 c	Tempeh Pâté, Tofu-Tempeh Lasagna	Basis of tempeh, tofu, and miso; good as extender in meat dishes; use in casseroles and spicy salads.
White (great northern, navy, small)	Round, large and small, mild taste, firm texture	6–7 c	1 hr	4 c	White Bean Soup, Marinated White Bean Salad, Meatless White Bean Bake	Shape holds up during cooking; use in soups and cassoulets.

ANGEL HAIR SAUTÉ

An elegant side dish. Pair it with a seafood entree such as Poached Salmon with Spinach Sauce (p. 263) and a fruit salad.

> 1 teaspoon margarine
> 2 tablespoons minced green onion
> 1 small clove garlic, minced
> 6 medium asparagus spears, cut into 1-inch pieces or ½ cup frozen asparagus spears
> ½ cup nonfat milk
> ¼ cup half-and-half
> 1 ounce Parmesan cheese, freshly grated
> 2 tablespoons light cream cheese
> ⅛ teaspoon white pepper
> 1 cup cooked angel hair pasta (cook according to package directions and keep warm)

1. In a large nonstick skillet, heat margarine, green onions, and garlic; sauté until tender, about 1 minute.
2. Add asparagus and cook, stirring occasionally until crisp-tender.
3. Stir in remaining ingredients, except pasta, and cook, stirring constantly, until mixture comes just to a boil.
4. Top pasta with sauce and serve.

Yield: 2 servings, 2 cups pasta, 1½ cups sauce
One Serving = 1 cup pasta, ¾ cup sauce

Calories: 169	Fiber: 1 g
Protein: 9 g	Cholesterol: 34 mg
Fat: 8 g	Sodium: 224 mg
Carbohydrate: 15 g	Potassium: 189 mg

Exchange: 1 starch/bread
1 medium-fat meat
½ fat

A favorite dish among Southwestern chefs, beans are increasing in popularity across the country. Top with yogurt or low-fat cheese to enhance flavor.

2 teaspoons vegetable oil	1 bay leaf
1 large onion, chopped	¼ teaspoon pepper
2 cloves garlic, minced	1 teaspoon white vinegar
1 green pepper, chopped	1 orange, unpeeled and halved
1 tomato, chopped	2 stalks celery, chopped
1 cup dried black beans	4 ounces lean ham or 8 ounces
3 cups chicken stock or water	ham hocks (optional)

1. Heat 2 teaspoons of oil in a large pot.
2. Sauté onion, garlic, green pepper, and tomato until soft.
3. Add beans, stock, bay leaf, and pepper. Bring to a boil, then reduce heat.
4. Simmer for 2 minutes and remove from stove.
5. Let sit, covered, for 1 hour.
6. Add vinegar, orange halves, and celery and cook 2 to 3 more hours until beans are tender.
7. Remove orange and bay leaf.
8. To thicken bean mixture, remove about ½ cup, mash, and return to pot.
9. For additional flavor, add 4 ounces of lean ham or 8 ounces of ham hocks.

Yield: 6 servings, 4½ cups (without ham)
One Serving = ¾ cup

Calories: 241	Fiber: 10.3 g*
Protein: 9 g	Cholesterol: 0
Fat: 10 g	Sodium: 27 mg†
Carbohydrate: 29 g	Potassium: 694 mg

Exchange: 2 starch/bread
             2 fat

*Good source of dietary fiber
†If you use ham, this is a high-sodium recipe.

CHEESY BROCCOLI AND PASTA _____

This easy side dish can be served as a summer luncheon entree.

   1 tablespoon vegetable oil or margarine
   1 cup diced onions
   1 cup diced red pepper
   1 clove garlic, minced
   1 tablespoon all-purpose flour
   1 package instant vegetable broth and seasoning mix
   1 cup nonfat milk
   ¼ cup blue cheese, crumbled
   3 tablespoons light cream cheese, whipped
   4 cups chopped broccoli florets, steamed
   3 cups cooked pasta (shells, macaroni, spirals, etc.)

1. In a large nonstick pot heat oil or margarine until hot; add onions, pepper, and garlic and sauté until onions are translucent.
2. Add flour and broth mix to onion mixture and stir quickly for about 1 minute; gradually add milk while continuing to stir. Bring to a boil.
3. Reduce heat to low; add cheeses and stir constantly until melted.
4. Fold in broccoli and cook until heated through. Serve over hot pasta.

Yield: 4 servings, 4 cups broccoli mixture and 3 cups pasta
One Serving = 1 cup broccoli mixture and ¾ cup pasta

   Calories: 182   Fiber: 2.3 g
   Protein: 8 g   Cholesterol: 9 mg
   Fat: 5 g   Sodium: 178 mg
   Carbohydrate: 26 g   Potassium: 361 mg

Exchange: 1 starch/bread
          2 vegetable
          1 fat

CHILI RICE

Serve with chicken for a spicy meal.

Rice

    1 teaspoon olive oil
    ½ onion, chopped
    2 cloves garlic, minced
    2 cups cooked brown rice

Sauce

    3 tablespoons salsa
    1 can (4 ounces) green chilies or 2 to 3 fresh Anaheim or California chilies
    ⅓ cup white vinegar
    ¼ cup chopped onion
    ½ cup chopped fresh cilantro

1. To prepare the rice, heat oil in a skillet. Add onion and garlic and sauté until onion is translucent.

2. Stir in cooked rice and heat thoroughly.

3. If using fresh chilies, grill or roast them by setting them under the broiler until they start to blister and turn brown. Turn chilies to broil evenly. Place chilies in a plastic bag and let steam 5 minutes or until cool. Remove from bag and peel skin using fingers or knife.

4. For the sauce, mix salsa, chilies, and vinegar in a blender or food processor.

5. Stir in onion and cilantro.

6. Pour chili sauce over rice and serve.

Yield: 4 servings, 3 cups
One Serving = ¾ cup (with fresh chilies)

Calories: 150
Protein: 3 g
Fat: 2 g
Carbohydrate: 31 g

Fiber: 2.5 g
Cholesterol: 0
Sodium: 382 mg (with 2 fresh jalapeño peppers)
Potassium: 203 mg

Exchange: 2 starch/bread

BULGUR PILAF _____ EASY

A great side dish to highlight any entree.

> **2 tablespoons margarine**
> **¾ cup bulgur wheat**
> **2 tablespoons chopped onion**
> **2 cups chicken broth**
> **Freshly ground black pepper to taste**

1. Melt margarine in large skillet and add bulgur and onion. Brown onion lightly, stirring often.
2. Add broth and bring to a boil; cover, reduce heat, and simmer for 15 to 20 minutes, or until the liquid is absorbed.
3. Season with pepper.

Yield: 6 servings, 3 cups
One Serving = ½ cup

Calories: 127	Fiber: 0.2 g
Protein: 4 g	Cholesterol: 0
Fat: 5 g	Sodium: 310 mg
Carbohydrate: 18 g	Potassium: 139 mg

Exchange: 1 starch/bread
            1 fat

FRIJOLES DE LA OLLA (BOILED MEXICAN BEANS) _ EASY

Beans from the pot that are simple and delicious!

> **1 pound pinto or pink beans**
> **5 cups water (or more)**
> **1 medium onion, diced**
> **1 teaspoon salt**

1. Rinse beans well. (Beans do not have to be soaked prior to cooking.) Place beans and onion in a large pot with the water. Cover and simmer over low heat for at least 3½ to 4 hours. (Alternatively, for overnight cooking, use a slow-cooker such as a Crockpot.)
2. Add the salt when the beans are done cooking.

Yield: 7 to 9 servings, 5 to 6 cups
One Serving = ⅔ cup

Calories: 158	Fiber: 5 g*
Protein: 10 g	Cholesterol: 0
Fat: <1 g	Sodium: 197 mg
Carbohydrate: 29 g	Potassium: 452 mg

Exchange: 2 starch/bread

*Good source of dietary fiber

FRIJOLES REFRITOS (REFRIED BEANS) ——————— QUICK

The name *refried beans* should not be taken literally. In Spanish, "re" sometimes means "very" or "thoroughly," so that one frying is enough.

2 tablespoons margarine
2½ cups cooked pinto beans with liquid (see recipe for Frijoles de la
    Olla, p. 198)
½ teaspoon salt
½ teaspoon cumin (optional)

1. Heat margarine in a frying pan.
2. Mash beans until fairly smooth.
3. Add beans to hot margarine and fry, scraping the pan to prevent sticking. Cook only until the beans are heated completely. Season with salt and cumin, if desired.

Yield: 4 servings, 2 cups
One Serving = ½ cup

Calories: 161	Fiber: 8.5 g*
Protein: 8 g	Cholesterol: 0
Fat: 5 g	Sodium: 220 mg
Carbohydrate: 22 g	Potassium: 487 mg

Exchange: 1½ starch/bread
         1 fat

*Good source of dietary fiber

INSALATA PASTA FREDDA (COLD PASTA SALAD) _____

This cold pasta salad tastes especially good the next day after the flavors have had a chance to blend.

1½ cups small shells or elbow macaroni, cooked
1 medium tomato, chopped
¼ cup diced onion
¼ cup diced green or red pepper
Cayenne pepper to taste
1 tablespoon chopped fresh cilantro
½ small clove garlic, minced
1 tablespoon olive oil
1½ teaspoons red wine vinegar
1½ teaspoons freshly squeezed lime juice
¼ teaspoon salt
⅛ teaspoon oregano
Dash of freshly ground black pepper

1. Combine pasta, tomato, onion, bell pepper, cayenne pepper, cilantro, and garlic in a large bowl.
2. In a small bowl, combine remaining ingredients; pour over salad and toss to coat. Cover and refrigerate until chilled. Stir before serving.

Yield: 4 servings, 4 cups
One Serving = 1 cup

Calories: 121
Protein: 3 g
Fat: 4 g
Carbohydrate: 19 g

Fiber: 1.2 g
Cholesterol: 0
Sodium: 137 mg
Potassium: 149 mg

Exchange: 1 starch/bread
          1 fat

MEATLESS WHITE BEAN BAKE

1½ cups navy beans or small white beans
1 cup canned tomatoes, drained
1 cup chicken broth
½ onion, finely chopped
2 cloves garlic, minced
½ teaspoon thyme
½ teaspoon salt
½ teaspoon freshly ground black pepper
¼ cup dry white wine (optional)

1. Wash the beans and soak overnight, or use the following shortcut: In a large pot, combine the beans with enough hot water to cover them plus 4 inches. Bring to a boil and boil for 2 minutes. Remove the pan from the heat. Let the beans soak for 1 hour and then drain.
2. In the same large pot, combine the beans with enough cold water to cover them plus 4 inches. Bring water to a boil, and simmer the beans for 40 to 60 minutes or until they are tender.
3. Preheat the oven to 300°F.
4. Combine the rest of the ingredients with the beans and stir. Bake, covered, in a casserole dish until the liquid is nearly absorbed, approximately 2 hours.

Yield: 6 servings, 4 cups
One Serving = ⅔ cup

Calories: 112
Protein: 7 g
Fat: <1 g
Carbohydrate: 20 g

Fiber: 4.4 g
Cholesterol: 0
Sodium: 312 mg
Potassium: 459 mg

Exchange: 1 starch/bread
         1 vegetable

MUESLI

Our version of a popular European breakfast cereal. Serve with non-fat milk or yogurt.

1 cup old-fashioned oats	⅓ cup chopped almonds
½ cup oat bran	¼ cup raisins
1½ cups plain low-fat yogurt	1 tablespoon honey
½ cup coarsely grated apple	1 teaspoon cinnamon
½ cup coarsely grated pear	½ teaspoon nutmeg

1. In a bowl, stir together the oats, oat bran, and yogurt.
2. Cover and chill mixture for 30 minutes.
3. Stir in apple, pear, almonds, raisins, honey, and spices.
4. Mix well.

Yield: 6 servings, 3 cups
One Serving = ½ cup

Calories: 216	Fiber: 3.8 g
Protein: 9 g	Cholesterol: 4 mg
Fat: 6 g	Sodium: 48 mg
Carbohydrate: 35 g	Potassium: 404 mg

Exchange: 2 starch/bread
        ½ fruit
        1 fat

PEPPERY PASTA

Low in calories but very flavorful; you can serve this special dish over your favorite pasta.

1 medium red pepper	1 tablespoon capers, drained
2 teaspoons olive oil	5 black olives, pitted and chopped
2 cloves garlic, minced	¼ teaspoon oregano
½ cup chopped canned tomatoes with liquid	2 cups cooked fettuccine

1. Roast pepper by charring under the broiler. Turn frequently to blacken all sides. Place inside a plastic bag and steam for 15 minutes.
2. Remove pepper from the bag and peel skin; remove ends and seeds; chop and set aside.

3. In a large nonstick skillet, heat oil and sauté garlic until browned.
4. Stir in tomatoes with liquid and cook 5 minutes.
5. Add roasted red pepper, capers, olives, and oregano.
6. Simmer until thoroughly heated, about 5 minutes.
7. Ladle sauce over pasta and serve.

Yield: 4 servings, 2 cups pasta, 1 cup sauce
One Serving = ½ cup pasta with ¼ cup sauce

Calories: 139	Fiber: 1.4 g
Protein: 4 g	Cholesterol: 25 mg
Fat: 4 g	Sodium: 102 mg
Carbohydrate: 22 g	Potassium: 146 mg

Exchange: 1 starch/bread
         1 vegetable
         1 fat

RED BEANS AND RICE _____ EASY

An ideal way to use leftover beans, rice, or ham.

2 cloves garlic, minced	**2 teaspoons Tabasco sauce**
⅓ cup diced onion	**2 cups cooked brown rice**
⅛ teaspoon each cayenne pepper,	**2 cups cooked red beans**
** cumin, and chili powder**	**1 cup diced cooked ham**

1. In a large pan, sauté garlic and onion with seasonings.
2. Add rice, beans, and ham; cook over medium heat.
3. Stir in approximately ¼ cup water or liquid from beans.
4. Cook until heated thoroughly.

Yield: 4 servings, 4 cups
One Serving = 1 cup

Calories: 306	Fiber: 10.4 g*
Protein: 19 g	Cholesterol: 21 mg
Fat: 4 g	Sodium: 555 mg†
Carbohydrate: 48 g	Potassium: 731 mg

Exchange: 3 starch/bread
         1 medium-fat meat

*Good source of dietary fiber
†High in sodium

SPANISH RICE

1 tablespoon margarine or vegetable oil
1 cup brown rice
5 green onions, chopped
1 medium tomato, chopped
¼ cup chopped green pepper
2 cups chicken broth, defatted
⅓ cup tomato juice
⅛ teaspoon chili powder

1. Heat margarine in a large nonstick skillet. Add rice and cook for 5 to 8 minutes.
2. Stir in remaining ingredients; cover and simmer for 45 minutes or until liquid is absorbed.

Yield: 8 servings, 6 cups
One Serving = ¾ cup

Calories: 90
Protein: 3 g
Fat: 3 g
Carbohydrate: 14 g

Fiber: 2.2 g
Cholesterol: <1 mg
Sodium: 233 mg
Potassium: 164 mg

Exchange: 1 starch/bread
½ fat

14

MEATLESS MAIN DISHES

MANY OF THESE DISHES may also be called vegetarian main dishes because they lack meat and feature protein from vegetables and grains. Many are ethnic in origin, borrowing from cultures all over the world that use meat sparingly — as a condiment or a way to flavor their plant-based dishes.

Try more meatless meals as you become accustomed to lowering your fat and cholesterol intake. Start off by trying meatless breakfasts and lunches and save your meat for the main course at dinner. Eventually you should be comfortable eating 2 to 3 meatless main meals per week.

Calzones
Crêpes, with Cheese-Herb or
   Sweet Cheese Filling
Chilaquiles
Delhi Delite
Falafel, with Tahini or Yogurt
   Dressing
Rice and Cheese Casserole

Pasta Pie Italiano
Pizza
Spaghetti Squash Casserole
Spicy Lentils with Cucumber
   Yogurt Dressing
Tofu-Tempeh Lasagna
Tricolor Squash Casserole
Zucchini Pie

CALZONES

These are rounds of yeast-raised dough, folded over and filled with a spinach-cheese mixture. Always a big hit!

Dough

> 2 teaspoons active dry yeast
> 1 tablespoon honey
> 1¼ cups warm water (110°F)
> 2 cups whole wheat flour
> 2 cups unbleached all-purpose flour
> ½ teaspoon salt (optional)
> Nonstick vegetable spray

Filling

> 1 pound fresh spinach (or two 10-ounce packages frozen spinach)
> 2 cloves garlic, crushed
> ½ cup minced onion
> 1 tablespoon olive oil
> 1 pound (2 cups) part-skim ricotta cheese
> 1 cup grated part-skim mozzarella cheese, or 1 cup pot, farmer, or low-fat cottage cheese
> ½ cup freshly grated Parmesan cheese
> Dash of nutmeg
> Salt and freshly ground black pepper to taste

1. Dissolve yeast and honey in water. Stir in flours and salt (if desired). Knead dough on a floured board for 10 to 15 minutes. Place in a bowl coated with nonstick spray, cover, and set in a warm place to rise until doubled in bulk (1 hour).
2. Punch the dough down. Divide into 8 sections and roll out into rounds approximately ¼ inch thick.
3. Wash, stem, and finely chop spinach. Steam it quickly over medium-high heat. It is done when wilted and deep green. Let it cool and squeeze out excess water. If using frozen spinach, let thaw. Then squeeze out excess water.
4. Sauté onion and garlic in olive oil until translucent and soft.
5. Combine all filling ingredients; mix well. Season with salt and pepper to taste.
6. Fill each dough round with ½ cup filling, placing filling on ½ circle and leaving a ½-inch rim. Moisten the rim with water, fold the empty side over, and crimp the edge with a fork.

7. Bake on a cookie sheet coated with nonstick spray in a preheated 450°F oven for 15 to 20 minutes, or until crisp and lightly browned.

Yield: 6 to 8 servings
One Serving = 1 calzone

Calories: 383	Fiber: 5.6 g*
Protein: 21 g	Cholesterol: 29 mg
Fat: 11 g	Sodium: 406 mg† (without
Carbohydrate: 52 g	salt)
	Potassium: 488 mg

Exchange: 3 starch/bread
            2 medium-fat meat

*Good source of dietary fiber
†High in sodium

CRÊPES

Adapted from *The New American Diet* by William and Sonja Connor.

This recipe is a low-fat, low-cholesterol version of the original, which calls for whole eggs, whole milk, and butter. You can fill a crêpe with almost anything. Try the Cheese-Herb Filling for a main dish at lunch or dinner. The Sweet Cheese Filling is good for brunch.

1 cup cold water	**½ teaspoon salt or less**
1 cup cold nonfat milk	**2 cups sifted all-purpose flour**
1 egg + 4 whites	**2 tablespoons vegetable oil**

1. Put liquids, egg, egg whites, and salt into blender; add flour, then oil. Blend at top speed, stopping to scrape flour from the sides.
2. Cover and refrigerate 2 hours. (This is an important step; it allows the flour particles to expand in the liquid and ensures a tender, thin crêpe. The batter should have a very light, creamy texture — just thick enough to coat a wooden spoon.)
3. For each crêpe, heat a 6-inch nonstick frying pan over moderately high heat. When hot, pour a scant ¼ cup of the batter into the skillet; immediately rotate pan until batter covers bottom. Cook until light brown; turn and brown other side. Slide onto a warm plate and proceed in the same manner with the rest of the batter.

4. Put waxed paper between the crêpes as you stack them.

5. Keep crêpes covered to prevent them from drying out. They are now ready to be filled.

Yield: 20 crêpes, 6 inches each
One Serving = 1 crêpe

Calories: 65	Fiber: 0.4 g
Protein: 3 g	Cholesterol: 14 mg
Fat: 2 g	Sodium: 47 mg
Carbohydrate: 10 g	Potassium: 44 mg

Exchange: 1 starch/bread

Serving, Storing, or Freezing of Crêpes
- Fill, fold, or roll and serve immediately.
- Prepare ahead. Pile up individually between layers of waxed paper. Wrap in foil, refrigerate, and reheat when ready to fill.
- Prepare in advance. Then freeze and reheat at the last minute. Wrap in heavy foil to freeze. They will keep for weeks.

Cheese-Herb Filling

1½ cups low-fat cottage or ricotta cheese	Salt and freshly ground black pepper to taste
1 green onion, minced	2 teaspoons margarine
Dash of basil	Tomato slices for garnish
Dash of chopped fresh parsley	

1. Mix cheese, onion, and herbs. Season with salt and pepper.

2. Fill each crêpe with 3 to 4 tablespoons of filling.

3. In a skillet over medium heat, lightly brown crêpes in margarine.

4. Garnish with tomato slices and serve.

Yield: 6 servings, 1½ cups
One Serving = ¼ cup

Calories: 63	Carbohydrate: 2 g	Sodium: 278 mg
Protein: 8 g	Fiber: 0.1 g	Potassium: 63 mg
Fat: 3 g	Cholesterol: 5 mg	

Exchange: 1 lean meat

Sweet Cheese Filling

This crêpe filling works equally well with blintzes. Serve them warm with fresh fruit toppings for a weekend breakfast.

¾ cup low-fat cottage cheese   ¼ teaspoon grated lemon peel
2 ounces Neufchâtel cheese   1 tablespoon margarine
2 teaspoons vanilla   ½ cup vanilla low-fat yogurt
2 teaspoons freshly squeezed   1 cup berries or sliced fruit in
    lemon juice   season

1. Prepare crêpes (recipe on p. 207). Set aside.
2. Blend cheeses, vanilla, lemon juice, and peel.
3. Fill each crêpe with ¼ cup mixture and roll.
4. In a nonstick skillet, sauté filled crêpes in margarine until slightly browned.
5. Top with low-fat yogurt and sliced fruit.

Yield: 4 servings, 1 cup filling
One Serving = ¼ cup filling plus yogurt-fruit topping

Calories: 160   Carbohydrate: 14 g   Sodium: 282 mg
Protein: 8 g   Fiber: 1.5 g   Potassium: 162 mg
Fat: 8 g   Cholesterol: 16 mg

Exchange: 1 lean meat
          1 fruit
          1 fat

CHILAQUILES _____

In Mexico this dish is usually eaten for breakfast. You may also enjoy it as a side dish for lunch or dinner.

18 corn tortillas	1 tablespoon vegetable oil
1½ pounds tomatillos	½ onion, chopped
2 to 3 cloves garlic	2 cups nonfat plain yogurt or 8
4 to 5 chiles serranos	ounces shredded low-fat cheese
¼ cup water or less	or 4 cups vegetarian refried beans

1. Prepare tortillas as in the No-Fry Tortilla Chips, p. 111.
2. Combine the tomatillos, garlic, and chiles in the water. Boil until the tomatillos soften and become darker.
3. Purée the ingredients in blender or food processor.
4. Warm the oil in a saucepan and add the blended mixture.
5. Stir the tortilla chips into the mixture until chips soften.
6. Serve hot, garnished with chopped onion and one of the remaining toppings.

Yield: 8 servings, 6 cups
One Serving = ¾ cup

	Without Topping	Yogurt	Cheese	Beans
Calories	152	186	231	287
Protein	5 g	8 g	13 g	13 g
Fat	4 g	4 g	9 g	5 g
Carbohydrate	27 g	32 g	28 g	51 g
Fiber	2.4 g	2.4 g	2.4 g	8 g*
Cholesterol	0	1 mg	28 mg	0
Sodium	353 mg	399 mg	235 mg	536 mg†
Potassium	349 mg	505 mg	376 mg	846 mg
Exchange:	1½ starch/bread 1½ vegetable 1 fat	1½ starch/bread 1½ vegetable 1 fat	1½ starch/bread 1 medium-fat meat 1½ vegetable	2½ starch/bread 1½ vegetable 1 fat

*Good source of dietary fiber
†High in sodium

DELHI DELITE

Rice is a staple in many cultures and is the basis for many vegetarian dishes. You can substitute turmeric for the saffron.

2 tablespoons margarine
2 teaspoons cumin seed or ¼ teaspoon ground cumin
¼ teaspoon salt
⅛ teaspoon cayenne pepper
2 tablespoons mustard seed (black or brown)
6 cups assorted, chopped fresh vegetables
¼ teaspoon saffron
Juice of 1 or 2 lemons (approximately ¼ to ½ cup)
6 cups cooked rice
⅓ cup slivered almonds
⅓ cup chopped raw, unsalted cashews
⅓ cup raisins
1 pint plain low-fat yogurt

1. Melt margarine with cumin, salt, cayenne, and mustard seed in a large skillet. Add vegetables and toss to coat with spices.
2. Cover and simmer until nearly tender.
3. Meanwhile, prepare saffron rice by dissolving saffron in lemon juice, then stirring in 3 cups cooked rice. Mix thoroughly.
4. In a 9 × 13-inch dish, layer as follows:
> plain boiled rice
> cooked vegetables
> saffron rice
> thin layer of nuts and raisins
> yogurt.

Repeat.
5. Bake covered for 40 minutes in a preheated 325°F oven.

Yield: 12 servings, 12 cups
One Serving = 1 cup

Calories: 251
Protein: 8 g
Fat: 7 g
Carbohydrate: 40 g
Exchange: 2 starch/bread
         2 vegetable
         1 fat

Fiber: 3.1 g
Cholesterol: 2.5 mg
Sodium: 95 mg
Potassium: 396 mg

FALAFEL

A spicy meatless entree — originally published in *The New American Diet* by William and Sonja Connor.

2 cups garbanzo beans, cooked, drained, and rinsed
⅓ cup water
1 slice crustless firm wheat bread, torn into pieces
1 tablespoon unbleached all-purpose flour
½ teaspoon baking soda
3 cloves garlic, finely chopped
1 egg white
2 tablespoons chopped fresh parsley
½ teaspoon salt
¼ teaspoon freshly ground black pepper
¼ teaspoon cumin
½ teaspoon turmeric
¼ teaspoon basil
¼ teaspoon marjoram
1 tablespoon tahini (sesame seed paste) or olive oil
Cayenne pepper to taste
Flour for coating the falafel

1. Purée the garbanzos in a food processor or in a blender.
2. Add the remaining ingredients, except the flour, and mix well. The mixture will be soft.
3. Form the mixture into 1-inch balls or patties and coat with flour.
4. Bake in a preheated 350°F oven for 15 to 20 minutes.
5. To make a falafel sandwich, cut a piece of pita bread in half and put 2 to 3 falafel balls or patties into the open halves. Add lettuce, alfalfa sprouts, sliced tomatoes, green onions, and low-fat Yogurt Dressing or Tahini Dressing (recipes follow).

Yield: 5 servings, 20 balls
One Serving = 4 balls

Calories: 158	Fiber: 3.3 g
Protein: 7 g	Cholesterol: 0
Fat: 5 g	Sodium: 341 mg
Carbohydrate: 23 g	Potassium: 237 mg

Exchange: 1½ starch/bread
           ½ medium-fat meat

Tahini Dressing
>   ¼ cup tahini (sesame seed paste)
>   ½ cup water or more
>   1 tablespoon freshly squeezed lemon juice
>   1 clove garlic, crushed

1. Mix all ingredients.
2. The mixture should be the consistency of a creamy salad dressing. Add more water if necessary.
3. Use as a sauce for a falafel sandwich.

Yield: 12 servings, ¾ cup
One Serving = 1 tablespoon

Calories: 31	Fiber: 0.4 g
Protein: 1 g	Cholesterol: 0
Fat: 3 g	Sodium: 4 mg
Carbohydrate: 1 g	Potassium: 30 mg

Exchange: 1 fat

Yogurt Dressing
>   1 cup plain nonfat yogurt
>   1 tablespoon freshly squeezed lemon juice
>   ⅛ teaspoon salt
>   1 tablespoon chopped fresh parsley

1. Combine all ingredients and serve with falafel.

Yield: 4 servings, 1 cup
One Serving = 4 tablespoons

Calories: 40	Fiber: <1 g
Protein: 3.5 g	Cholesterol: 0
Fat: 1 g	Sodium: 111 mg
Carbohydrate: 4.5 g	Potassium: 152 mg

Exchange: ½ nonfat milk

RICE AND CHEESE CASSEROLE ———————————— EASY

Easy to prepare, this recipe is very high in calcium.

> 2½ cups cooked brown rice
> 3 green onions, chopped
> 1 cup low-fat cottage cheese
> 1 teaspoon dill weed
> ¼ cup freshly grated Parmesan cheese
> ½ cup low-fat milk
> ½ teaspoon Dijon-style mustard
> Nonstick vegetable spray

1. Combine all but the last ingredient in a mixing bowl.
2. Pour into a casserole dish coated with nonstick vegetable spray.
3. Bake in a preheated 350°F oven for 15 to 20 minutes.

Yield: 6 servings, 4 cups
One Serving = ¾ cup

Calories: 225	Fiber: 2.5 g
Protein: 14 g	Cholesterol: 10 mg
Fat: 4 g	Sodium: 328 mg
Carbohydrate: 34 g	Potassium: 218 mg

Exchange: 1½ starch/bread
½ lean meat
1 low-fat milk

PASTA PIE ITALIANO ————————————————

A novel way to serve spaghetti.

Crust
> 2 cups cooked spaghetti
> 2 egg whites
> 1 tablespoon freshly grated Parmesan cheese
> Nonstick vegetable spray

Topping

    ¼ onion, sliced

    ½ pound zucchini, thinly sliced

    1 clove garlic, minced

    7 ounces chopped tomatoes (approximately 2 medium)

    ½ cup tomato sauce

    ¼ teaspoon oregano

    ¼ teaspoon basil

    1 cup part-skim ricotta cheese

    3 egg whites

    ¼ cup nonfat milk

    4 ounces part-skim mozzarella cheese, freshly grated

    ¼ cup freshly grated Parmesan cheese

1. Preheat oven to 375°F.

2. Combine spaghetti, egg whites, and 1 tablespoon Parmesan cheese and press into a 9-inch pie plate coated with nonstick spray.

3. Cook onion and zucchini in microwave or in a nonstick pan until soft.

4. Cook garlic, tomatoes, tomato sauce, and seasonings in a saucepan to reduce by half. Set aside.

5. Spoon zucchini mixture into the bottom of the pie shell.

6. Pour ¼ of the tomato mixture over the pie.

7. Blend ricotta with egg whites and milk and spoon over top of pie. Bake for 40 minutes.

8. Spread with remaining tomato mixture and top with mozzarella and Parmesan. Bake 7 to 8 minutes longer.

Yield: 6 servings, 1 9-inch pie
One Serving = ⅙ pie

    Calories: 234   Fiber: 1.7 g

    Protein: 17 g   Cholesterol: 26 mg

    Fat: 8 g   Sodium: 394 mg

    Carbohydrate: 22 g   Potassium: 405 mg

Exchange: 1 starch/bread
            2 medium-fat meat
            1 vegetable

Here are two variations of homemade pizza. Add one of our suggested pizza toppings to make a lower-fat version of traditional pizza.

Yeast Crust
This recipe makes one thin crust.

> **1 teaspoon active dry yeast**
> **½ teaspoon honey**
> **½ cup warm water (110°F)**
> **¼ teaspoon salt (optional)**
> **½ tablespoon olive oil**
> **1¼ cups unbleached all-purpose flour or ¾ cup wheat flour + ½ cup unbleached all-purpose flour**
> **Nonstick vegetable spray**

1. Preheat oven to 350°F.
2. In a medium bowl, dissolve yeast and honey in water. Let stand until bubbly, about 5 to 10 minutes.
3. Add salt (if desired), oil, and ½ cup flour. Stir thoroughly.
4. Add remaining flour gradually. As dough thickens, mix flour in with hands.
5. Turn dough onto lightly floured surface and knead until smooth and elastic, about 5 minutes. Place dough in bowl coated with nonstick spray, cover, and let rise in a warm, draft-free area for about 45 minutes.
6. Punch down dough and knead again for several minutes on a lightly floured surface.
7. Roll out dough to fit a 12-inch pizza pan. Coat pan with nonstick spray. Spread dough onto pan.
8. Place toppings on pizza, beginning with tomato sauce, and bake in top third of oven for 10 to 12 minutes or until crust is golden and cheese has melted.

Yield: 8 servings
One Serving = 1 slice

Calories: 74	Fiber: 0.3 g
Protein: 2 g	Cholesterol: 0
Fat: <1 g	Sodium: 62 mg
Carbohydrate: 14 g	Potassium: 27 mg

Exchange: 1 starch/bread

Beer Batter Crust

This quick and easy recipe makes a thick, Sicilian-style square crust. Credit for this recipe goes to the authors of *The New American Diet,* William and Sonja Connor.

2 cups unbleached all-purpose flour	1 tablespoon baking powder
1 cup whole wheat flour	12 ounces beer
	Nonstick vegetable spray

1. In a large bowl mix all ingredients. Spread evenly into a 9 × 13-inch pan coated with nonstick spray.
2. Sprinkle with one of the toppings from pp. 217–219.
3. Bake in a preheated 425°F oven for 25 to 30 minutes or until done.

Yield: 12 pieces
One Serving = 3 × 3-inch square

Calories: 113
Protein: 3 g
Fat: <1 g
Carbohydrate: 23 g

Fiber: 1.3 g
Cholesterol: 0
Sodium: 87 mg
Potassium: 67 mg

Exchange: 1½ starch/bread

Cheesy Topping

1 cup tomato sauce
¾ cup part-skim ricotta cheese
½ ounces Romano cheese, freshly grated
2 ounces part-skim mozzarella cheese, freshly grated
2 cloves garlic, minced
1 cup sliced mushrooms
Oregano and basil

	Yeast Crust, Cheesy Topping:	Beer Crust, Cheesy Topping:
Calories	145	161
Protein	8 g	7 g
Fat	5 g	3 g
Carbohydrate	19 g	26 g
Fiber	0.5 g	0.4 g
Cholesterol	13 mg	9 mg
Sodium	284 mg	267 mg
Potassium	208 mg	162 mg

Exchange: 1 starch/bread   1½ starch/bread
1 medium-fat meat   ½ medium-fat meat

Greek Topping

 1 cup tomato sauce

 Fresh spinach

 1 cup crumbled feta cheese

 20 black olives, pitted and sliced

 1 cup sliced or diced tomato

	Yeast Crust, Greek Topping:	*Beer Crust, Greek Topping:*
Calories	154	158
Protein	6 g	5 g
Fat	7 g	4 g
Carbohydrate	19 g	26 g
Fiber	1 g	1.7 g
Cholesterol	17 mg	8 mg
Sodium	471 mg*	354 mg
Potassium	237 mg	169 mg

Exchange: 1 starch/bread
          1 vegetable
          1 fat

1 starch/bread
1½ vegetable
1 fat

Vegetarian Topping

 1 cup tomato sauce

 2 cups assorted vegetables, chopped and steamed

 ¼ cup freshly grated Parmesan cheese

	Yeast Crust, Vegetarian Topping:	*Beer Crust, Vegetarian Topping:*
Calories	125	147
Protein	5 g	5 g
Fat	2 g	1 g
Carbohydrate	23 g	28 g
Fiber	1.4 g	2 g
Cholesterol	2 mg	2 mg
Sodium	321 mg	260 mg
Potassium	221 mg	196 mg

Exchange: 1 starch/bread
          2 vegetable

1 starch/bread
½ medium-fat meat
½ vegetable

*High in sodium

Basic Italian Topping
  1 cup tomato sauce
  1 cup freshly grated low-fat mozzarella cheese
  1 cup sliced mushrooms
  1 green pepper, sliced
  Oregano and basil

	Yeast Crust, Italian Topping:	*Beer Crust, Italian Topping:*
Calories	150	165
Protein	6 g	6 g
Fat	5 g	3 g
Carbohydrate	20 g	27 g
Fiber	0.6 g	1.5 g
Cholesterol	8 mg	5 mg
Sodium	284 mg	235 mg
Potassium	197 mg	201 mg

Exchange:	1 starch/bread	1 starch/bread
	1 vegetable	2 vegetable
	1 fat	½ medium-fat meat

SPAGHETTI SQUASH CASSEROLE ———————— MICROWAVE

Spaghetti squash is a lower-calorie alternative to pasta. Its mild flavor makes it ideal for use with a variety of sauces or seasonings.

> **1 8-inch-long spaghetti squash**
> **1 cup chopped onion**
> **2 to 3 cloves garlic, crushed**
> **1 tablespoon olive oil**
> **1 cup sliced mushrooms**
> **1½ teaspoons basil**
> **1 teaspoon oregano**
> **⅛ teaspoon thyme**
> **2 tomatoes, chopped**
> **Nonstick vegetable spray**
> **½ cup part-skim ricotta cheese**
> **¼ cup freshly grated part-skim mozzarella cheese**
> **¼ cup freshly chopped parsley**
> **1 cup whole wheat bread crumbs**
> **2 tablespoons freshly grated Parmesan cheese**

1. Preheat oven to 375°F. Slice squash in half lengthwise and scoop out seeds. Pierce shell and place in baking pan. Bake uncovered, face down, for 30 minutes. Turn squash over and continue to bake for about 20 more minutes, until softened. When cool, remove spaghetti strands with a fork.

2. While the squash bakes, sauté the onion and garlic in the olive oil with the mushrooms and herbs. When onions are soft, add tomatoes. Cook until most of the liquid evaporates.

3. Remove mixture from stove and pour into a 2-quart casserole that has been coated with nonstick vegetable spray.

4. Stir in ricotta, mozzarella, parsley, bread crumbs and cooked squash.

5. Sprinkle with Parmesan cheese and bake, uncovered, at 375°F for 30 to 40 minutes, until cheese is browned.

Microwave

1. Slice the squash in half lengthwise and scoop out the seeds. Place the squash, hollow side up, on a flat 12-inch plate. Cover with plastic wrap. Cook in microwave on High for 8 to 10 minutes, rotating dish ¼ turn after 5 minutes. Squash should be fork-tender when pierced. Set aside. When cool, scoop out insides.

2. In a casserole dish, combine onion, garlic, oil, and mushrooms. Cover with waxed paper and cook on high for 3 to 4 minutes. Add herbs and tomatoes. Cook uncovered, 2 to 3 minutes more, until slightly thickened and juice from the tomatoes has evaporated. Let stand for 5 minutes.

3. Add the ricotta, mozzarella, parsley, and bread crumbs to the casserole dish and top with Parmesan. Cook uncovered for 6 to 8 minutes on high. Squash should retain a slightly crunchy consistency.

Yield: 6 servings, 6 cups
One Serving = 1 cup

Calories: 227	Fiber: 7 g
Protein: 9 g	Cholesterol: 10 mg
Fat: 7 g	Sodium: 197 mg
Carbohydrate: 34 g	Potassium: 557 mg

Exchange: 2½ vegetable
½ low-fat milk
1 fat
1 starch/bread

SPICY LENTILS WITH CUCUMBER YOGURT DRESSING —

An ethnic dish from India. The cool, creamy Cucumber Yogurt Dressing complements the spicy lentils.

Spicy Lentils
- 1½ cups lentils
- 2¼ cups water
- 1 teaspoon olive oil
- 2 cloves garlic, crushed
- 1 cup minced onion
- 1 stalk celery, finely chopped (½ cup)
- ½ teaspoon salt (optional)
- ½ teaspoon ginger
- ½ teaspoon turmeric
- ½ teaspoon cinnamon
- ½ teaspoon curry powder
- ½ teaspoon coriander
- ½ cup raisins
- Juice of a large lemon
- 2 cups chopped Granny Smith apples (or other tart apple)
- Red and freshly ground black pepper, to taste

Cucumber Yogurt Dressing
- 2 cups plain low- or nonfat yogurt
- 2 cucumbers, coarsely grated
- 1 tablespoon white wine vinegar
- ½ teaspoon salt
- 1 tablespoon dill weed
- ½ teaspoon cumin
- 2 to 3 cloves garlic, crushed and minced

1. Place lentils in a saucepan and cover with 2¼ cups of water. Bring to a boil, cover, reduce heat, and simmer for about 45 minutes.

2. In a deep skillet, heat olive oil. Sauté garlic, onion, celery, seasonings, raisins, and lemon juice until tender. Add a tablespoon of water if mixture becomes too dry.

3. Add apples to vegetable mixture, cover, and cook for 10 minutes over low heat.

4. Combine apple-vegetable mixture with lentils. Place in a casserole dish.

5. In a bowl, combine all the ingredients for the Cucumber Yogurt Dressing. Serve with the Spicy Lentils and pita bread.

Yield for lentils: 8 to 10 servings
One Serving = 1 cup

Calories: 139	Fiber: 5.5 g*
Protein: 7 g	Cholesterol: 0
Fat: 1 g	Sodium: 154 mg
Carbohydrate: 29 g	Potassium: 358 mg

Exchange: 2 starch/bread

Yield for dressing: 8 servings, 4 cups
One Serving = ½ cup

Calories: 49	Fiber: 0.9 g
Protein: 4 g	Cholesterol: 0
Fat: 1 g	Sodium: 178 mg
Carbohydrate: 7 g	Potassium: 244 mg

Exchange: ½ nonfat milk

*Good source of dietary fiber

TOFU-TEMPEH LASAGNA

Not as heavy as meat-cheese lasagna, yet a filling and delicious crowd pleaser, especially for the vegetarian. Low-sodium tomato sauce really decreases the sodium content of this dish.

    10 to 12 ounces lasagna noodles
    10 to 12 ounces tempeh
    2 tablespoons olive oil
    1 medium onion, diced
    1 medium green pepper, diced
    1 to 2 cloves garlic, minced
    4 to 6 teaspoons chopped fresh oregano or 2 to 3 teaspoons dried
    4 to 6 teaspoons chopped fresh basil or 2 to 3 teaspoons dried
    3 to 4 cups tomato sauce (low-sodium)
    1 pound fresh spinach or 2 packages (10 ounces each) frozen chopped
        spinach, thawed
    1 pound tofu
    ½ teaspoon salt (optional)
    1 cup freshly grated part-skim mozzarella cheese
    1 large tomato, sliced

1. Cook noodles in boiling water until tender, 12 to 15 minutes. Rinse in cool water and drain on paper towels.
2. Cut tempeh into ¼-inch cubes and sauté in olive oil until browned. Add onion, pepper, and garlic. Brown an additional 5 minutes. Add oregano, basil, tomato sauce, and simmer 10 to 15 minutes more. Set aside.
3. Wash, drain, and chop fresh spinach. Steam, in water clinging to its leaves, until wilted and deep green (or thaw frozen chopped spinach).
4. Drain tofu well and mash with a fork. Stir in salt, if desired, and spinach.
5. Layer in a lightly oiled 9 × 12-inch baking dish as follows: a third of the noodles, half of the tofu mixture, and a third of the tempeh-tomato sauce; repeat, then the remaining noodles and the remaining sauce; then the cheese and the tomato slices.
6. Bake in a preheated 350°F oven for 20 to 25 minutes or until cheese is browned on top.

Yield: 8 servings
One Serving = approximately 1 cup

Calories: 430
Protein: 26 g
Fat: 13 g
Carbohydrate: 58 g

Fiber: 3.6 g
Cholesterol: 9 mg
Sodium: 292 mg (without salt)
Potassium: 1133 mg

Exchange: 3 starch/bread
2 medium-fat meat
2 vegetable

TRICOLOR SQUASH CASSEROLE

A very colorful dish! Serve with rice or pasta to balance out the meal.

Tomato Sauce
> 1 tablespoon olive oil
> 4 cloves garlic, minced
> 2 onions, diced
> 4 cups peeled and chopped tomatoes
> 2 tablespoons tomato paste
> ¼ cup minced fresh basil leaves
> ½ teaspoon salt (optional)
> ¼ teaspoon freshly ground black pepper

> Nonstick vegetable spray
> 4 large zucchini, sliced into ⅛-inch-thick pieces
> 6 ounces part-skim mozzarella cheese, shredded
> 6 ounces part-skim Monterey Jack cheese, shredded
> 4 large pattypan squash, sliced into ⅛-inch-thick pieces
> 4 large crookneck squash, sliced into ⅛-inch-thick pieces
> ¼ cup freshly grated Parmesan cheese

1. Combine all ingredients for tomato sauce in a blender and purée.
2. Lightly coat a 13 × 9-inch baking pan with nonstick vegetable spray. Cover with sliced zucchini. Spoon ¼ cup of the tomato sauce over the zucchini and sprinkle with ⅓ of the mozzarella cheese and ⅓ of the Monterey Jack cheese.
3. Arrange pattypan squash over the cheese and spoon ½ of the remaining tomato sauce over the squash. Sprinkle with another ⅓ of the mozzarella and Jack cheeses.
4. Arrange crookneck squash over the cheese and cover with the remaining mozzarella and Jack. Top with remaining tomato sauce and sprinkle with Parmesan. Season with salt, if desired, and pepper.
5. Bake in a preheated 375°F oven for 30 to 40 minutes or until squash is tender and cheese is melted.

Yield: 8 servings, 8 cups
One Serving = 1 cup

Calories: 255
Protein: 18 g
Fat: 14 g
Carbohydrate: 21 g

Fiber: 6.5 g*
Cholesterol: 34 mg
Sodium: 345 mg (without salt)
Potassium: 1345 mg

Exchange: 2 medium-fat meat
4 vegetable
½ fat

*Good source of dietary fiber

ZUCCHINI PIE

This recipe is courtesy of William and Sonja Connor, authors of *The New American Diet*.

Crust

    1 tablespoon active dry yeast
    ½ cup warm water (110°F)
    ½ cup whole wheat flour
    ¾ cup unbleached all-purpose flour
    ¼ teaspoon salt
    Nonstick vegetable spray

Filling

    4 cups thinly sliced zucchini
    1 cup coarsely chopped onion
    1 tablespoon margarine
    2 tablespoons chopped fresh parsley
    ½ teaspoon freshly ground black pepper
    ¼ teaspoon garlic powder
    ¼ teaspoon sweet basil
    ¼ teaspoon oregano
    2 eggs or 4 egg whites
    2 cups freshly grated part-skim mozzarella cheese
    2 teaspoons Dijon-style mustard

1. Dissolve yeast in water. Stir in flours and salt. Knead dough on floured board for 5 minutes or until smooth and elastic. Turn into a bowl coated with nonstick spray, cover, and let rise for 45 minutes in a warm, draft-free area.

2. In a large skillet, cook zucchini and onion in margarine until tender, about 10 minutes. Stir in parsley and seasonings.

3. In a large bowl, blend eggs and cheese. Stir in vegetable mixture.

4. Transfer raised dough to an ungreased 11-inch quiche pan, 10-inch pie pan, or 9 × 13-inch baking dish; press over bottom and up sides to form crust. Spread crust with mustard. Pour vegetable mixture evenly into crust.

5. Bake in a preheated 375°F oven for 25 to 35 minutes or until knife inserted near center comes out clean. If crust becomes too brown, cover with foil during the last 10 minutes of baking. Let stand 10 minutes before serving.

Yield: 6 servings
One Serving = ⅙ pie

Calories: 261
Protein: 17 g
Fat: 11 g
Carbohydrate: 25 g

Fiber: 3 g
Cholesterol: 112 mg
Sodium: 359 mg
Potassium: 403 mg

Exchange: 1 starch/bread
2 medium-fat meat
1 vegetable

15

MEAT, POULTRY, AND SEAFOOD

AMERICANS are making a transition: we are eating smaller portions of meat, fish, and poultry than we used to because of the high saturated fat and cholesterol content of these foods. The days of the 18-ounce steak and country-fried half chicken are becoming less and less common. Our recipes offer some interesting and healthful alternatives that will become an integral part of your new eating plan.

Beef, veal, and lamb are important sources of vitamins and minerals — namely, zinc, iron, and magnesium. In small amounts these meats can contribute significantly to the nutritional quality of your diet. The diet for the 1990s is one that includes lean meat in moderation. Our recipes should give you new and different ideas as to how to use meat as a "condiment" or as a complement to vegetables and grains (such as the moussaka or cassoulet).

Poultry has been promoted as a lower-fat alternative to beef, yet some poultry recipes can have *twice* as many calories and fat if not chosen wisely! This is particularly true of fried chicken and chicken prepared in heavy cream sauces. Think light! Poultry without skin (most of the fat and saturated fat is in the skin) and dishes that feature light-meat poultry are low in fat and reduced in calories. You can combine ground turkey, a relative newcomer to the market, with a variety of delicious seasonings and sauces. It makes for a perfect beef substitute from burgers to meat loaf.

It is also important to incorporate seafood into your new, lighter style of eating. Most types of seafood are lower in calories, saturated fat, total fat, and cholesterol, so everyone can enjoy them. Seafood

230

is also an excellent source of vitamins A, D, and B-complex, and is particularly rich in the omega-3 fatty acids. You can prepare fish in the microwave, in the oven, or on the grill. Try including some type of fish as a main dish in your daily diet *at least* twice a week.

Beef and Bean Chili
Beef Stroganoff
Beef with Oyster Sauce
Cassoulet
Beef Roulade
Grilled Onion Burgers
One-Pan Spaghetti
Kabobs
Pork Chops à l'Orange
Pork with Red Chili Sauce
Veal Parmesan
Vegetable Meat Loaf

BBQ Chicken
Cheese and Broccoli–Stuffed
  Chicken
Chicken Adobo
Chicken Artichoke Pie
Chicken Breasts Dijon
Chicken Italiano
Chicken Marsala with
  Mushrooms
Chicken with Forty Cloves of
  Garlic

Herb-Roasted Chicken
Ginger Chicken
Grilled Game Hens
Spicy Thai Chicken
Mediterranean Moussaka
Parmesan Chicken
Turkey Loaf

Baked Halibut with Cilantro-
  Citrus Sauce
Basic Blackened Catfish
Crab Cakes
Fish Fillets Provençale
Fish Tacos
Poached Salmon with Spinach
  Sauce
Lemony Shrimp Curry
Roulade of Sole
Shellfish and Artichoke
  Casserole
Shrimp and Feta with Tofu
Shrimp with Cashews
Snapper Creole
Teriyaki Fish Fillets

BEEF AND BEAN CHILI _____

Top this chili with a few dollops of nonfat yogurt, a sprinkling of freshly grated low-fat cheese, or some chopped onions.

½ pound pinto beans
1 onion, chopped
1 green pepper, chopped
1 pound extra lean ground beef (or ground turkey)
2 to 3 cloves garlic, minced
1 tablespoon chili powder
2 teaspoons cumin
2 teaspoons cayenne pepper (optional)
1 can (28 ounces) tomatoes, drained
1 can (6 ounces) tomato sauce

1. Add pinto beans to a 1-quart saucepan and cover them with water. Cook over medium heat 1 hour or until tender.
2. Simmer onion and green pepper in ¼ cup water in a large nonstick skillet until onion is translucent.
3. Add ground beef and cook over medium heat until browned.
4. Drain excess fat from pan.
5. Stir in garlic, chili powder, cumin, and cayenne (for spicier taste).
6. Add drained tomatoes, tomato sauce, and beans to chili mixture.
7. Stir well and simmer, uncovered, for 15 minutes.
8. Cover and cook for ½ hour over low heat.

Yield: 6 servings, 6 cups
One Serving = 1 cup

Calories: 311
Protein: 23 g
Fat: 11 g
Carbohydrate: 33 g

Fiber: 4.8 g
Cholesterol: 47 mg
Sodium: 443 mg*
Potassium: 1065 mg

Exchange: 2 starch/bread
3 lean meat

*High in sodium

BEEF STROGANOFF _____

This dish is a lower-fat, lower-calorie rendition of the all-time classic.

> 1½ pounds beef round steak, cut ½ inch thick and trimmed of fat
> 1 tablespoon olive oil
> 2 cups sliced mushrooms
> ½ cup dry sherry
> ½ cup water
> ½ teaspoon instant beef bouillon granules
> 8 ounces plain low-fat yogurt
> 1 tablespoon all-purpose flour
> ¼ teaspoon salt
> Dash of black pepper
> 5⅓ cups hot cooked rice or 8 cups noodles
> Chopped fresh parsley (optional)

1. Thinly slice steak across the grain into bite-size strips. Heat olive oil in skillet and brown meat, half at a time, in the hot oil for 2 to 4 minutes. Remove meat from the skillet.

2. Add sliced mushrooms to the skillet and cook for 2 to 3 minutes or until tender. Remove mushrooms.

3. Add sherry, water, and bouillon granules to skillet; bring to boiling. Cook, uncovered, over high heat, about 3 minutes or until liquid is reduced.

4. Combine yogurt, flour, salt, and pepper; mix well.

5. Stir yogurt mixture into liquid in skillet; add meat and mushrooms. Cook and stir over low heat until thickened and heated through. Do not boil.

6. Serve over rice or noodles. Sprinkle the stroganoff mixture with snipped parsley, if desired.

Yield: 8 servings, 4 cups
One Serving = ½ cup sauce with 1 cup rice or noodles

Calories: 322	Fiber: 1.5 g
Protein: 26 g	Cholesterol: 65 mg
Fat: 9 g	Sodium: 198 mg
Carbohydrate: 31 g	Potassium: 433 mg

Exchange: 2 starch/bread
           3 lean meat

BEEF WITH OYSTER SAUCE

This dish works well as an entree, served with rice and stir-fried vegetables, or as a hot appetizer.

1 pound boneless lean beef (flank or sirloin)
6 green onions, sliced
2 tablespoons soy sauce
1 tablespoon cornstarch
1 tablespoon oil
2 tablespoons oyster sauce

1. Cut beef into thin slices.
2. Combine onions, soy sauce, 3 tablespoons water, and cornstarch.
3. Pour over meat and marinate for 10 to 15 minutes.
4. Heat a wok or a large skillet; add oil when hot.
5. Add meat mixture, stirring quickly to cook. (You may find it easier to cook half at a time.)
6. Add oyster sauce and cook 1 minute longer. Add water if necessary to prevent sticking.

Yield: 4 servings, 2 cups
One Serving = ½ cup

Calories: 246	Fiber: trace
Protein: 27 g	Cholesterol: 76 mg
Fat: 13 g	Sodium: 571 mg*
Carbohydrate: 3 g	Potassium: 394 mg

Exchange: 3 lean meat
          1 fat
          1 vegetable

*High in sodium

CASSOULET

Serve this modification of the French country classic with crusty Parmesan Herb Bread (p. 184). The slow cooking melds the full flavors of this timeless recipe.

1 cup navy beans
4 cups cold water
3 cups hot water
½ cup chopped onion
½ cup chopped celery
½ cup chopped carrot
1 teaspoon instant chicken bouillon granules
¼ pound boneless lean lamb, cut into ½-inch cubes
½ cup diced cooked ham
1 bay leaf
3 tablespoons dry white wine
1 teaspoon Worcestershire sauce
1 teaspoon chopped fresh basil or ½ teaspoon dried
1 teaspoon chopped fresh oregano or ½ teaspoon dried

1. Rinse beans well. In a large saucepan, combine beans and cold water. Bring to a boil; reduce heat. Cover and simmer for 2 minutes. Remove from heat. Cover and let stand for 1 hour. (Or soak beans in 4 cups cold water overnight in covered pan.) Drain beans and rinse.
2. In the same saucepan, combine the rinsed beans, hot water, onion, celery, carrots, and bouillon. Cover and simmer for 30 minutes.
3. Add lamb, ham, and bay leaf. Simmer, covered, for 30 minutes more.
4. Remove bay leaf. Stir in wine, Worcestershire sauce, basil, and oregano.
5. Turn mixture into a 2-quart casserole. Cover and bake in a pre-heated 350°F oven for 45 minutes. Uncover and bake for 40 to 45 minutes more, stirring occasionally.

Yield: 4 servings, 4 cups
One Serving = 1 cup

Calories: 166
Protein: 14 g
Fat: 6 g
Carbohydrate: 15 g

Fiber: 5.3 g*
Cholesterol: 30 mg
Sodium: 466 mg†
Potassium: 530 mg

Exchange: 1 starch/bread
1½ lean meat

*Good source of dietary fiber
†High in sodium

BEEF ROULADE _____

2 pounds lean sirloin roast
1 medium onion, thinly sliced
3 dill pickles, thinly sliced
   lengthwise

6 strips bacon
1 cup Burgundy or other red wine
2 to 3 black peppercorns
1 bay leaf

1. Trim all visible fat from the roast. Slice into 6 very thin, 3 × 3-inch pieces.
2. On top of each piece of meat, place onion slices, then 1 to 2 pickle strips, followed by 1 strip of bacon.
3. Starting at one end, roll the meat tightly and fasten with a toothpick. Place meat in a Dutch oven or saucepan.
4. Add wine, peppercorns, bay leaf, and enough water to barely cover meat.
5. Cover and bake in a preheated 325°F oven for 1½ hours — or, if using a saucepan, simmer gently for the same amount of time.
6. Check every 30 to 45 minutes; turn meat and add more water if necessary to prevent meat from drying out. Turn meat at this time.

Yield: 6 servings
One Serving = 4 ounces

Calories: 222
Protein: 28 g
Fat: 11 g
Carbohydrate: 2 g

Fiber: 1 g
Cholesterol: 72 mg
Sodium: 346 mg
Potassium: 428 mg

Exchange: 4 lean meat

GRILLED ONION BURGERS _____ EASY, MICROWAVE

Try these burgers with ground turkey instead of ground beef, for less fat and fewer calories.

¼ cup dry white wine
2 tablespoons chopped fresh basil
½ cup chopped onion
1 pound leanest ground beef (10 percent fat)
4 whole wheat buns
Burger condiments

1. Combine ingredients and refrigerate for 1 hour or more.
2. Shape into 4 patties and grill or cook on the stove.
3. Serve on whole wheat buns with your favorite condiments.

Microwave
Cook patties 3 minutes per side or until desired doneness.

Yield: 4 servings, 4 burgers
One Serving = 1 burger, 3 ounces

Calories: 344 (with bun)	Fiber: 0.5 g
Protein: 26 g	Cholesterol: 71 mg
Fat: 16 g	Sodium: 301 mg
Carbohydrate: 23 g	Potassium: 406 mg

Exchange: 3 medium-fat meat
    2 bread

ONE-PAN SPAGHETTI _____ EASY

An easily prepared dish for children.

½ pound leanest ground beef (10 percent fat)

2 cups water

2 cups spaghetti sauce (meatless, low-sodium)

½ cup chopped onion

¼ cup chopped green pepper

½ teaspoon chili powder

1 teaspoon chopped garlic

1 teaspoon oregano

5 ounces spaghetti

2 tablespoons freshly grated Parmesan cheese

1. In a large skillet, combine ground beef, water, spaghetti sauce, onion, green pepper, chili powder, garlic, and oregano.
2. Bring to a boil. Reduce heat and simmer, covered, for 30 minutes. Stir often.
3. Add the spaghetti; simmer, covered, for 30 minutes. Stir often. Serve with Parmesan cheese.

Yield: 4 servings, 6 cups
One Serving = 1½ to 2 cups

Calories: 253	Fiber: 3.5 g
Protein: 15 g	Cholesterol: 24 mg
Fat: 7 g	Sodium: 83 mg
Carbohydrate: 33 g	Potassium: 664 mg

Exchange: 2 starch/bread
1½ lean meat
1 vegetable

KABOBS _____

Presoaking bamboo skewers in water prevents them from burning when broiling or grilling kabobs.

½ pound beef sirloin
½ cup herb wine vinegar
2 tablespoons vegetable oil
2 tablespoons chopped fresh parsley
½ teaspoon freshly ground black pepper
½ medium onion, cut into large chunks
1 green pepper, seeded and cut into wide strips
6 cherry tomatoes, halved
8 unsweetened pineapple chunks, drained

1. Trim fat from sirloin and cut meat into 1½-inch cubes.
2. Mix vinegar, oil, parsley, and pepper.
3. Marinate meat in mixture for approximately 2 hours, stirring occasionally.
4. Alternate meat on 4 skewers with onion, green pepper, tomatoes, and pineapple. Or skewer and cook meat and vegetable cubes separately to prevent excess browning.
5. Brush with marinade.
6. Broil 4 inches from heat for about 10 minutes or grill over a hot fire, turning to brown evenly.

Yield: 4 servings, 4 skewers
One Serving = 1 skewer

Calories: 205
Protein: 12 g
Fat: 13 g
Carbohydrate: 10 g

Fiber: 1.8 g
Cholesterol: 38 mg
Sodium: 24 mg
Potassium: 312 mg

Exchange: 2 lean meat
2 vegetable
1 fat

PORK CHOPS À L'ORANGE ───────────────

6 pork loin chops, trimmed of fat
1¼ cups orange juice
1 tablespoon cornstarch
1 orange, sliced, for garnish
Parsley sprigs for garnish

1. Place chops in a baking dish and cover with foil.
2. Bake in a preheated 350°F oven for 20 minutes.
3. Combine orange juice and cornstarch in a small bowl and pour over the chops.
4. Return chops to the oven, covered, and continue to bake 20 more minutes or until done.
5. Remove to a serving platter and garnish with orange slices and parsley.

Microwave
1. Place pork chops in baking dish with the thicker portion toward the outside of the dish.
2. Pour ¼ cup orange juice over meat. Cover tightly with plastic wrap and vent one corner.
3. Cook on high for 6 minutes per side.
4. Meanwhile, combine the remaining orange juice with cornstarch, mixing well. Pour this sauce over the chops.
5. Return to microwave and cook an additional 1 to 2 minutes on high until sauce is thickened.
6. Remove to a serving platter and spoon sauce over chops. Garnish with orange slices and parsley.

Yield: 6 chops
One Serving = 1 3-ounce chop

Calories: 233	Fiber: 0.2 g
Protein: 23 g	Cholesterol: 77 mg
Fat: 12 g	Sodium: 59 mg
Carbohydrate: 7 g	Potassium: 411 mg

Exchange: 3 medium-fat meat
           ½ fruit

PORK WITH RED CHILI SAUCE _____

Serve this traditional Mexican entree as a filling for corn or flour tortillas or as an accompaniment to rice and beans. Garnish with tomato slices and fresh cilantro for a colorful meal.

3 pounds boneless lean pork butt
2 tablespoons vegetable oil
2 large onions, chopped
2 cloves garlic, minced or pressed
6 teaspoons chili powder
1 teaspoon cumin
1½ teaspoons oregano
1¼ cups water
1 teaspoon honey
½ teaspoon salt
3 tablespoons tomato paste

1. Trim and discard all fat from the meat and cut into 1-inch cubes.
2. Heat oil in a large skillet over medium-high, and cook meat, a few pieces at a time, until brown.
3. Push meat to one side of the pan, add onion, garlic, chili powder, cumin, and oregano; cook until onion is limp.
4. Stir in water, honey, salt, and tomato paste. Simmer, covered, until pork is tender, about 1 hour. Skim off fat and discard.
5. To serve, fill warm corn or flour tortillas (made with margarine) with meat mixture. Include rice or beans, if desired, and garnish.

Yield: 6 servings, 3 cups
One Serving = ½ cup (4 ounces pork)

Calories: 329	Fiber: 1.6 g
Protein: 34 g	Cholesterol: 109 mg
Fat: 17 g	Sodium: 381 mg
Carbohydrate: 8 g	Potassium: 658 mg

Exchange: 4 medium-fat meat
          1 vegetable

VEAL PARMESAN _____

A healthful alternative to a classic dish.

> **1 pound veal leg round steak**
> **½ cup chopped onion**
> **1 clove garlic, minced**
> **¼ cup chopped green pepper**
> **2 teaspoons olive oil**
> **2 tablespoons freshly grated Parmesan cheese**
> **1 cup tomato sauce**
> **1 tablespoon dry red or white wine**
> **½ teaspoon Italian seasoning**
> **2 ounces freshly shredded part-skim mozzarella cheese**

1. Cut veal into 4 pieces; pound to ¼-inch thickness.
2. In a large skillet, cook onion, garlic, and green pepper in oil until tender. Push to one side of the skillet; add veal and brown on both sides.
3. Combine Parmesan cheese, tomato sauce, wine, and seasoning. Pour over meat and cover.
4. Cook over low heat for 20 to 25 minutes, or until meat is tender.
5. Sprinkle mozzarella cheese over meat. Cover for 1 to 2 minutes more to melt the cheese.

Yield: 4 servings
One Serving = 4 ounces meat and sauce

Calories: 240
Protein: 31 g
Fat: 10 g
Carbohydrate: 7 g

Fiber: 1.3 g
Cholesterol: 115 mg
Sodium: 694 mg*
Potassium: 523 mg

Exchange: 4 lean meat
           1 vegetable

*High in sodium

VEGETABLE MEAT LOAF

This recipe is almost an entire meal by itself! The vegetables make the loaf moist and lower the fat content.

4 cups finely shredded cabbage (about 1 pound)
½ cup finely chopped onion
1 tablespoon vegetable oil
1 cup shredded carrots, firmly packed
2 medium or 1 large clove garlic, minced (about 1 heaping teaspoon)
½ pound lean ground round (10 to 15 percent fat)
3 egg whites
⅓ cup bread crumbs
1 teaspoon basil
½ teaspoon oregano
½ teaspoon salt or less
¼ to ½ teaspoon freshly ground black pepper
¼ cup water
2 tablespoons white vinegar
1 cup shredded potatoes, firmly packed

1. In a large skillet, sauté the cabbage and onion in the oil over medium heat for approximately 5 minutes. Stir often; add 1 or 2 tablespoons water if the vegetables begin to stick. Reduce the heat to low and cook 5 to 10 minutes longer or until the cabbage begins to turn golden.
2. Add the carrots and garlic and sauté another 5 minutes. Remove the vegetables from the heat and allow them to cool to room temperature.
3. In a bowl, combine beef, egg whites, bread crumbs, basil, oregano, salt, pepper, water, and vinegar. Add the cooked vegetables and shredded potatoes. Mix well.
4. In a shallow baking pan, shape the mixture into a loaf. Cover the pan tightly with aluminum foil.
5. Bake the meat loaf in a preheated 350°F oven for 30 minutes. Uncover the loaf and bake an additional 30 minutes. Let the meat loaf rest for 15 minutes before slicing.

Yield: 8 servings
One Serving = ⅛ loaf

Calories: 145
Protein: 10 g
Fat: 7 g
Carbohydrate: 12 g

Fiber: 1.8 g
Cholesterol: 24 mg
Sodium: 185 mg
Potassium: 387 mg

Exchange: 1 lean meat
          2 vegetable
          1 fat

BBQ CHICKEN ———————————————— MICROWAVE

A summertime favorite — serve with Confetti Corn (p. 158) and Fresh Fruit Kabobs (p. 281).

4 chicken breast halves, skinned
1 clove garlic, chopped
1 bay leaf
½ cup barbecue sauce

1. In a large pot, place chicken, garlic, bay leaf, and enough water to cover.
2. Bring to a boil. Then gently simmer for 30 minutes.
3. Transfer chicken to a large plate.
4. Brush chicken liberally with sauce.
5. Grill 5 to 10 minutes per side or until done.
6. Brush on additional sauce as needed.

Microwave
1. Rub chicken with whole garlic clove. (Omit bay leaf.)
2. Cook chicken in microwave, covered with a glass lid or waxed paper, on high for approximately 10 minutes. Turn over chicken pieces after first 5 minutes.
3. Remove from microwave and let stand 10 minutes.
4. Continue with steps 4, 5, and 6 of the basic recipe.

Yield: 4 servings
One Serving = 1 chicken breast half, 3 ounces

Calories: 178
Protein: 27 g
Fat: 4 g
Carbohydrate: 7 g

Fiber: 0.3 g
Cholesterol: 66 mg
Sodium: 321 mg
Potassium: 327 mg

Exchange: 3 lean meat
          1 vegetable

CHEESE AND BROCCOLI–STUFFED CHICKEN _____

A variation of the classic Chicken Cordon Bleu, lower in fat and calories with a vegetable substitute. Try asparagus or spinach for the filling.

½ cup freshly grated low-fat cheese (mozzarella, Monterey Jack, or
    Swiss)
¼ cup diced onion
½ cup finely chopped broccoli
4 chicken breasts, skinned, boned, flattened, and rinsed
2 tablespoons fine bread crumbs
1 tablespoon sesame seeds
1 tablespoon chopped fresh parsley or ½ teaspoon dried
¼ teaspoon freshly ground black pepper
½ teaspoon paprika
Nonstick vegetable spray

1. Combine cheese, onion, and broccoli in a bowl.
2. Drop about 1 tablespoon of this mixture onto the largest end of each chicken breast.
3. Roll up and seal with toothpicks, making sure both sides are tucked in.
4. Combine bread crumbs, sesame seeds, parsley, pepper, and paprika for breading in a shallow pan.
5. Roll the chicken breasts in the mixture to coat evenly.
6. Arrange in a rimmed baking dish that has been coated with nonstick vegetable spray.
7. Bake in a preheated 350°F oven, uncovered, for approximately 40 minutes or until done.

Yield: 4 servings, 4 breasts
One Serving = 1 breast, 3 ounces

Calories: 198	Fiber: 0.8 g
Protein: 31 g	Cholesterol: 69 mg
Fat: 6 g	Sodium: 174 mg
Carbohydrate: 4 g	Potassium: 329 mg

Exchange: 3 lean meat
          1 vegetable

CHICKEN ADOBO ———————————————— EASY

Let the chicken marinate overnight to enhance the flavors of this unusual dish. Serve with rice.

4 chicken breast halves, skinned
2 large cloves garlic, crushed
1 medium onion, chopped
½ cup rice vinegar
¼ cup low-sodium soy sauce
¼ cup water
2 bay leaves
1 teaspoon sugar
⅛ teaspoon freshly ground black pepper

1. Rinse chicken pieces and place in a large pot.
2. Mix the remaining ingredients and pour over chicken to cover.
3. Cover the pot and simmer chicken for about 1 hour or until the chicken is very tender.
4. Remove bay leaves and serve with a small amount of marinade.

Yield: 4 servings
One Serving = 3-ounce piece chicken

Calories: 171	Fiber: 1 g
Protein: 29 g	Cholesterol: 72 mg
Fat: 3 g	Sodium: 544 mg*
Carbohydrate: 8 g	Potassium: 381 mg

Exchange: 3 lean meat

*High in sodium

CHICKEN ARTICHOKE PIE _____

Practically a complete meal. Top it off with Fruit Medley (p. 284) for dessert.

    1 package (10 ounces) frozen chopped spinach
    2 cups cooked white or brown rice
    1 tablespoon margarine, softened
    1 package (9 ounces) frozen artichoke hearts, thawed
    1½ cups cooked, skinned, and diced chicken
    1 cup freshly shredded part-skim mozzarella cheese
    ¼ pound mushrooms

"Cream" Sauce
    1 tablespoon margarine
    2 tablespoons all-purpose flour
    ½ teaspoon curry powder
    ½ teaspoon garlic powder
    1 teaspoon Dijon-style mustard
    1 cup nonfat milk
    Salt and freshly ground black pepper

1. Cook spinach according to package directions. Drain well and squeeze out all liquid.

2. Combine spinach and rice. Mix in margarine and press onto the bottom and sides of a 9-inch pie pan. Cover and chill for 30 minutes to 1 hour.

3. Drain artichokes; cut each into 2 to 3 pieces. Arrange over rice. Layer chicken, then cheese and mushrooms.

4. Combine all the ingredients for the sauce and pour over the spinach mixture. (The casserole may be refrigerated at this point.) Bake in a preheated 350°F oven for 1 hour or until bubbly.

Yield: 6 servings
One Serving = ⅙ pie

Calories: 286
Protein: 21 g
Fat: 10 g
Carbohydrate: 29 g

Fiber: 4.3 g
Cholesterol: 40 mg
Sodium: 300 mg
Potassium: 520 mg

Exchange: 1 starch/bread
           3 lean meat
           2 vegetable

CHICKEN BREASTS DIJON

A favorite among our taste testers! Serve the chicken with sauce over rice or noodles.

½ cup all-purpose flour
1 teaspoon paprika
4 chicken breasts, skinned and boned
1 tablespoon vegetable oil
1 cup chicken broth, refrigerated and then defatted
2 tablespoons Dijon-style mustard
3 cloves garlic, minced (more if desired)
2 green onions, finely chopped
Fresh parsley for garnish

1. In a paper or plastic bag, mix flour and paprika.
2. Drop chicken breasts (one at a time) into bag, shake, and remove.
3. Put oil in an ovenproof baking dish and place in preheated 350°F oven until hot.
4. Add chicken pieces to dish and bake for 20 minutes.
5. In a separate bowl, blend chicken broth with mustard and garlic.
6. After 20 minutes, turn chicken breasts and pour broth mixture over them.
7. Sprinkle with half of the green onions and bake another 20 minutes until done.
8. Garnish with the remaining green onions and parsley.

Yield: 4 servings
One Serving = 1 breast, 4 ounces

Calories: 305
Protein: 40 g
Fat: 9 g
Carbohydrate: 13 g

Fiber: 1 g
Cholesterol: 93 mg
Sodium: 378 mg
Potassium: 460 mg

Exchange: 1 starch/bread
         4 lean meat

A robust Italian country dish.

  1 3- to 3½-pound chicken, cut into pieces, skinned
  Salt and freshly ground black pepper (optional)
  1 tablespoon olive oil
  2 carrots, peeled and cut into ¼-inch-thick rounds
  2 stalks celery, cut into ¼-inch pieces
  3 cloves garlic
  2 cups dry white wine
  ¼ cup white wine vinegar
  ½ cup Chicken Stock (p. 290) or canned broth
  1 6-inch whole dried red chili
  1 small lemon, halved and seeded
  7 to 8 fresh sage leaves or ⅛ teaspoon dried
  3 fresh thyme sprigs or ⅛ teaspoon dried
  3 fresh rosemary sprigs or 1½ teaspoons dried

1. Preheat oven to 350°F and bake chicken pieces in the oven for approximately 20 minutes or until partially done. Season with salt and pepper if desired, and set aside.

2. Measure olive oil into a large Dutch oven. Add carrots and celery and sauté for 3 minutes. Add garlic and stir 1 minute. Add wine and vinegar and bring to a boil.

3. Add stock and chili to the sauce. Then squeeze juice from the lemon into the sauce; add the lemon halves. Bring back to a boil, reduce heat, and simmer for 15 minutes.

4. Add chicken legs and thighs to the Dutch oven. Increase the heat to medium and cook, covered, for 8 minutes. Add the remaining chicken pieces, sage, thyme, and rosemary, and cook until all the chicken is tender, stirring occasionally, about 15 to 20 minutes.

5. Adjust seasonings; discard the chili and lemon rinds. Garnish with remaining thyme sprigs and serve.

Microwave

1. Cook chicken parts in microwave, covered with a glass lid or waxed paper, on high for approximately 7 minutes. It is best to stop after 3½ minutes to turn over the wings and drumsticks, then restart the microwave.

2. Make the sauté and sauce according to directions outlined in steps 2 and 3 of the basic recipe.

3. Place chicken pieces in an 8 × 12-inch casserole dish suitable for a microwave. Pour sauce over chicken.
4. Add sage, thyme, and rosemary and cook in the microwave, covered, for 3 minutes. Uncover, stir, and baste chicken with sauce. Cook, covered, for 3 to 5 more minutes, or until chicken is done.
5. Serve from casserole dish, spooning sauce over chicken.

Yield: 4 servings, 8 pieces of chicken
One Serving = 2 small chicken pieces, 4 ounces with vegetables

Calories: 258	Fiber: 2.3 g
Protein: 35 g	Cholesterol: 94 mg
Fat: 11 g	Sodium: 286 mg
Carbohydrate: 5 g	Potassium: 613 mg

Exchange: 4 lean meat
           1 vegetable

CHICKEN MARSALA WITH MUSHROOMS _____

The Marsala wine provides a wonderful aroma while this dish is cooking. Serve with pasta and a salad.

- **1 tablespoon margarine**
- **2 green onions, chopped**
- **2 cloves garlic, crushed**
- **10 to 15 large mushrooms, sliced**
- **½ cup dry Marsala wine (or extra-dry sherry)**
- **2 tablespoons all-purpose flour**
- **4 chicken breast halves, skinned, boned, and flattened to ¼ inch thick**

1. In a large nonstick skillet, melt the margarine and sauté the onion, garlic, and mushrooms until soft.
2. Stir in ¼ cup wine and simmer for 5 minutes.
3. Meanwhile, spoon flour into a plastic bag.
4. One by one, shake the chicken breasts in the bag until the meat is lightly coated.
5. Return chicken to skillet and brown, approximately 4 minutes on each side, over medium heat.
6. Add the remaining wine and simmer for 10 to 15 minutes or until chicken is tender.

Yield: 4 servings
One Serving = 1 chicken breast half, 4 ounces

Calories: 254
Protein: 37 g
Fat: 8 g
Carbohydrate: 8 g

Fiber: 2.3 g
Cholesterol: 87 mg
Sodium: 118 mg
Potassium: 705 mg

Exchange: 4 lean meat
1 vegetable

CHICKEN WITH FORTY CLOVES OF GARLIC _____ EASY

Our version of a classic French country dish.

1 frying chicken, cut in pieces and skinned
40 cloves fresh garlic, unpeeled
½ cup dry white wine
½ cup dry vermouth
2 tablespoons olive oil
4 stalks celery, cut in 1-inch pieces
1 teaspoon oregano
2 teaspoons basil
2 tablespoons minced fresh parsley
Pinch of crushed red pepper
1 lemon
Salt and freshly ground black pepper to taste

1. Preheat oven to 350°F.
2. Place chicken pieces in shallow baking dish and sprinkle the next 9 ingredients evenly over top of chicken.
3. Squeeze juice from lemon and pour over top. Cut remaining lemon rind into pieces and scatter over chicken. Season with salt and pepper.
4. Cover with foil and bake for 40 minutes. Remove foil and baste chicken with its juice. Bake an additional 15 minutes.

Yield: 6 servings
One Serving = 4 ounces

Calories: 199
Protein: 25 g
Fat: 10 g
Carbohydrate: 1 g

Fiber: 0.3 g
Cholesterol: 71 mg
Sodium: 73 mg
Potassium: 262 mg

Exchange: 4 lean meat

A 3- to 5-pound chicken is called a roaster, but you can cook small broiler-fryers this way too.

2½- to 5-pound chicken
½ to 1 ounce fresh herbs (thyme, rosemary, marjoram, mint, or a combination of your favorites)

1. Preheat oven to 325°F. Rinse and pat chicken dry, removing organ meats and neck from the cavity.
2. Cut a small slit in the skin on each side of the breast of the chicken, or simply peel back the skin. Spread half of the herbs under the skin of the chicken on each side. Any leftover herbs can be placed in the cavity of the chicken for additional flavor.
3. Cook the chicken about 25 minutes for each pound, or approximately 1½ hours.
4. Remove from oven and let stand for 10 minutes before carving.
5. Remove skin before serving.

Yield: 4 to 6 servings
One Serving = 4 ounces

Calories: 215
Protein: 33 g
Fat: 8 g
Carbohydrate: 0

Fiber: 0.8 g
Cholesterol: 94 mg
Sodium: 95 mg
Potassium: 353 mg

Exchange: 4 lean meat

GINGER CHICKEN ———————————— EASY, MICROWAVE

Serve with rice or noodles and a vegetable stir-fry.

4 chicken breasts, split, skinned, and boned

Ginger Sauce
- **1 teaspoon ginger**
- **1 teaspoon vegetable oil**
- **4 green onions, finely chopped**
- **2 cloves garlic, finely chopped**
- **2 tablespoons low-sodium soy sauce**
- **3 tablespoons oyster sauce**
- **2 tablespoons water**

1. Preheat oven to 350°F.
2. Place chicken breasts in a shallow baking pan and bake for 10 minutes.
3. Combine ingredients for ginger sauce and pour over the chicken breasts.
4. Bake for an additional 15 minutes or until done.

Microwave
1. Place the chicken breasts in a microwave-safe dish and cook on high for 5 minutes.
2. Combine ginger sauce ingredients and pour over the chicken.
3. Cook on high for an additional 2 to 3 minutes.

Yield: 4 servings
One Serving = 1 chicken breast, 3 ounces

Calories: 163	Fiber: 0.6 g
Protein: 27 g	Cholesterol: 65 mg
Fat: 4 g	Sodium: 302 mg
Carbohydrate: 2 g	Potassium: 361 mg

Exchange: 3 lean meat

GRILLED GAME HENS _____ EASY

2 Cornish game hens (1½ pounds each)

Marinade

 1 cup freshly squeezed lemon juice
 ½ onion, chopped
 2 cloves garlic, minced
 1 tablespoon Worcestershire sauce
 1 teaspoon Tabasco sauce
 1 tablespoon freshly ground black pepper

1. Place hens breast side up and, with a sharp knife, cut through the top of the breast bone. Spread apart and press to flatten. Place hens in a pan large enough to accommodate them in 1 layer.

2. Combine marinade ingredients well and pour over hens; cover with plastic wrap.

3. Allow hens to marinate for 8 to 24 hours.

4. Remove hens from pan and grill them over hot coals (about 4 inches from heat).

5. Turn hens several times and cook approximately 20 minutes or until done.

Yield: 4 servings
One Serving = ½ game hen, approximately 4 ounces

Calories: 198	Fiber: 1 g
Protein: 29 g	Cholesterol: 86 mg
Fat: 8 g	Sodium: 188 mg
Carbohydrate: 4 g	Potassium: 562 mg

Exchange: 4 lean meat

SPICY THAI CHICKEN _____

A perfect accompaniment to brown or white rice. This recipe can easily be doubled.

½ small red bell pepper, chopped
2 tablespoons white vinegar
¼ teaspoon red pepper flakes
1 package Equal
2 chicken breasts, skinned
Lime wedges for garnish

1. Purée red pepper with vinegar in a blender or food processor.
2. Pour into a saucepan, add red pepper flakes, and bring the mixture to a boil.
3. Reduce to a simmer and cook for 3 minutes.
4. Remove from the heat and let the sauce cool.
5. When cooled, stir in the Equal.
6. Broil chicken breasts for 10 minutes or until browned; turn chicken and broil approximately 5 minutes more.
7. Place each chicken breast on a bed of rice. Divide spicy sauce and ladle over the top of the chicken.
8. Garnish with lime wedges and serve.

Yield: 2 servings
One Serving = 1 chicken breast, 4 ounces

Calories: 195
Protein: 35 g
Fat: 4 g
Carbohydrate: 2 g

Fiber: 0.2 g
Cholesterol: 87 mg
Sodium: 81 mg
Potassium: 355 mg

Exchange: 4 lean meat

MEDITERRANEAN MOUSSAKA _____

Serve with bread, rice, or pasta, and fresh vegetables.

    2 medium eggplants
    Lemon juice, to prevent discoloration
    2 tablespoons olive oil
    1 large onion, finely chopped
    3 cloves garlic, minced
    ½ pound leanest ground lamb
    ½ pound ground turkey
    10 fresh mushrooms, sliced
    1 can (8 ounces) tomato sauce
    1 large tomato, chopped
    1 bay leaf
    ¼ teaspoon Beau Monde seasoning (optional)
    1 tablespoon chopped fresh oregano or ¼ teaspoon dried
    Freshly ground black pepper to taste
    ½ cup dry red wine
    1 cup low-fat cottage cheese
    ½ teaspoon cinnamon
    ½ teaspoon allspice
    ¼ cup freshly grated Parmesan cheese
    2 tablespoons chopped fresh parsley

1. Peel eggplant and cut into ½-inch slices. To eliminate excess moisture, stack the slices in a colander or on paper towels, cover with a plate, place a heavy weight on top, and let stand until moisture is squeezed out. Rub the eggplant with lemon juice to keep it from discoloring.

2. Arrange half of the eggplant slices in the bottom of a 9 × 13 × 2-inch baking pan.

3. Heat olive oil in a large skillet and cook onion and garlic over medium heat until golden. Add meats and cook, stirring, for about 5 minutes, breaking up any lumps. Add mushrooms and sauté for 3 to 5 minutes more.

4. In a saucepan, heat tomato sauce, tomato, bay leaf, Beau Monde (if desired), oregano, and pepper. Cook for 10 minutes over medium heat. Add red wine and set aside.

5. Arrange the chopped meat mixture over the eggplant slices.

6. Mix the cottage cheese, cinnamon, and allspice, and sprinkle over the meat.

7. Cover the casserole with the remaining eggplant slices and pour the tomato sauce mixture over all. Sprinkle with Parmesan cheese.
8. Bake for 1 hour in a preheated 350°F oven until the top is golden. Remove from the oven and sprinkle with chopped parsley.

Yield: 6 servings, 6 cups
One Serving = 1 cup

Calories: 268
Protein: 25 g
Fat: 12 g
Carbohydrate: 17 g

Fiber: 4.5 g
Cholesterol: 55 mg
Sodium: 282 mg
Potassium: 872 mg

Exchange: 1 medium-fat meat
2 lean meat
3 vegetable

PARMESAN CHICKEN ——————————— MICROWAVE

1 onion, diced
1 cup diced celery
4 chicken breast halves, skinned and boned
1 cup tomato sauce or spaghetti sauce
¼ cup red wine
1 tablespoon Italian seasoning
1 tablespoon freshly grated Parmesan cheese

1. In a covered microwave-safe casserole, cook onion and celery in microwave until tender, 1 to 2 minutes on high. Remove from dish and set aside.
2. Place chicken in casserole, cover, and cook for 5 minutes on high.
3. Combine tomato sauce with wine and seasonings; pour over chicken and cook for 1 to 2 minutes longer.
4. Add cooked onion and celery to the chicken. Sprinkle Parmesan cheese over top; cook an additional 1 to 2 minutes.

Yield: 4 chicken breast halves
One Serving = 1 chicken breast, 3 ounces

Calories: 226
Protein: 30 g
Fat: 6 g
Carbohydrate: 13 g

Fiber: 2 g
Cholesterol: 75 mg
Sodium: 575 mg*
Potassium: 742 mg

Exchange: 3 lean meat
           2 vegetable

*High in sodium

TURKEY LOAF _____ EASY

A lower-fat version of traditional meat loaf — lean ground turkey replaces the usual ground beef.

>**1 egg, lightly beaten**
>**¼ cup bread crumbs**
>**2 tablespoons snipped fresh parsley**
>**½ teaspoon poultry seasoning**
>**1 teaspoon Dijon-style mustard**
>**¼ teaspoon freshly ground black pepper**
>**1 tablespoon chopped fresh basil (optional)**
>**1 pound ground turkey**
>**¼ cup chopped onion**

Sauce
>**1 tablespoon nonfat or low-fat yogurt**
>**2 teaspoons Dijon-style mustard**

1. In a bowl, combine egg, bread crumbs, parsley, poultry seasoning, mustard, pepper, and basil, if desired. Add turkey and onion; mix well.

2. Press evenly into an ungreased 8 × 5-inch loaf pan.

3. Bake in a 350°F oven for 35 minutes or until done.

4. Mix sauce ingredients and spread over top before serving.

Yield: 5 servings
One Serving = 3 ounces

Calories: 169
Protein: 22 g
Fat: 6 g
Carbohydrate: 6 g

Fiber: 0.5 g
Cholesterol: 112 mg
Sodium: 146 mg
Potassium: 268 mg

Exchange: 2½ lean meat
          1 vegetable

BAKED HALIBUT WITH CILANTRO-CITRUS SAUCE — EASY

Full of flavor, a Southern California favorite.

2 pounds halibut steaks or other firm fish steaks
½ cup chopped onion
2 cloves garlic, minced
1 tablespoon vegetable oil
2 tablespoons chopped fresh cilantro
⅛ teaspoon freshly ground black pepper
½ cup orange juice
1 tablespoon freshly squeezed lemon juice

1. Arrange fish in a shallow baking dish.
2. In a nonstick skillet, sauté onion and garlic in oil until tender. Add cilantro and pepper.
3. Stir in orange juice and lemon juice; pour over fish.
4. Bake, covered, in a preheated 400°F oven for 20 to 25 minutes or until fish flakes.

Yield: 6 servings
One Serving = 4 ounces

Calories: 160
Protein: 28 g
Fat: 3 g
Carbohydrate: 3 g

Fiber: 0.2 g
Cholesterol: 77 mg
Sodium: 120 mg
Potassium: 441 mg

Exchange: 4 lean meat

BASIC BLACKENED CATFISH ———————————— QUICK

A Cajun specialty with a lower fat content than the classic southern dish.

1 tablespoon olive oil
1 tablespoon Worcestershire sauce
2 catfish fillets, 8 ounces each

1 to 2 tablespoons Cajun Spice
(p. 291)
1 lemon, halved and seeded

1. Preheat broiler.
2. Mix olive oil and Worcestershire sauce. Baste fillets with mixture. Sprinkle Cajun Spice on top of fillets. Squeeze lemon juice over all.

3. Broil for 2 to 3 minutes, turn, repeat step 2, and broil 1 to 2 minutes more or until done.

Yield: 4 servings
One Serving = 3 ounces

Calories: 154	Fiber: 0
Protein: 22 g	Cholesterol: 62 mg
Fat: 6 g	Sodium: 64 mg
Carbohydrate: <1 g	Potassium: 565 mg

Exchange: 3 lean meat

CRAB CAKES ———————————————————— EASY

An Eastern seafood favorite.

½ cup crushed saltine crackers (approximately 10 saltines)
1 cup crabmeat
1 stalk celery, chopped
1 tablespoon diced onion
1 egg
2 teaspoons margarine
Tabasco sauce

1. Combine all ingredients except margarine and Tabasco in a bowl and mix until well blended.
2. Form 4 patties using ¼ of the mixture for each.
3. Melt margarine in a large nonstick skillet and fry patties until lightly browned, turning once.
4. Top each patty with a splash of Tabasco sauce.

Yield: 4 patties
One Serving = 1 patty

Calories: 111	Fiber: 0.6 g
Protein: 9 g	Cholesterol: 105 mg
Fat: 5 g	Sodium: 223 mg
Carbohydrate: 7 g	Potassium: 169 mg

Exchange: 1 lean meat
        1 starch/bread

FISH FILLETS PROVENÇALE _____ EASY

1 cup dry white wine
1 clove garlic, crushed
1 teaspoon oregano
¼ teaspoon thyme
4 6-ounce fish fillets (halibut, red snapper, or sea bass)
1 can (16 ounces) tomatoes or 3 fresh tomatoes, chopped
1 small onion, chopped

1. Combine wine, garlic, oregano, and thyme.
2. Place fillets in a baking dish.
3. Cover with tomato and onion.
4. Pour wine sauce over fish.
5. Cover and bake in a preheated 350°F oven for 30 to 35 minutes.

Yield: 4 fillets
One Serving = 1 fillet

Calories: 236	Fiber: 1.7 g
Protein: 32 g	Cholesterol: 56 mg
Fat: 9 g	Sodium: 75 mg
Carbohydrate: 6 g	Potassium: 834 mg

Exchange: 4 lean meat
         1 vegetable

FISH TACOS _____ QUICK

A tasty dish from South of the Border. Try adding low-fat cheese or your favorite vegetables for variety.

½ cup nonfat milk
¾ cup seasoned bread crumbs
8 ounces firm fish fillets (red snapper, sea bass, etc.)
Nonstick vegetable spray
8 corn tortillas
1 cup shredded cabbage
1 tomato, sliced
Tartar sauce, or salsa and fresh cilantro (optional)

1. Pour milk into one shallow pan and bread crumbs into another.
2. Gently coat fish by dipping first into milk, then into crumbs. Be sure that the fish is completely coated.
3. Place fillets on a baking sheet that has been coated with nonstick spray and bake in a preheated 350°F oven for 10 minutes or until fish is done.
4. Warm the corn tortillas in the oven and place the fillets, cabbage, and tomato slices on top.
5. Serve with tartar sauce or salsa and fresh cilantro, if desired.

Yield: 8 tacos
One Serving = 1 taco

Calories: 118	Fiber: 1.7 g
Protein: 9 g	Cholesterol: 11 mg
Fat: 2 g	Sodium: 104 mg
Carbohydrate: 17 g	Potassium: 260 mg

Exchange: 1 starch/bread
          1 lean meat

POACHED SALMON WITH SPINACH SAUCE _____

1 cup water
1 pound salmon steak

1. Bring 1 cup water to a boil in a medium skillet.
2. Add salmon and bring to a simmer. Cover and simmer for 5 minutes.
3. Carefully turn salmon over and cook for approximately 5 minutes more or until done.
4. Arrange on a platter and serve with Spinach Sauce (p. 264).

Yield: 4 servings
One Serving = 3 ounces

Calories: 134	Fiber: 0
Protein: 23 g	Cholesterol: 65 mg
Fat: 4 g	Sodium: 31 mg
Carbohydrate: 0	Potassium: 564 mg

Exchange: 3 lean meat

SPINACH SAUCE _____ EASY

Serve as a sauce over your favorite grilled or poached fish.

**1 pound fresh spinach, cleaned and stemmed, or 10 ounces frozen,
   chopped or leaves**
2 tablespoons margarine
2 tablespoons all-purpose flour
Freshly ground black pepper to taste
Pinch of nutmeg
1 cup nonfat plain yogurt at room temperature
¼ cup low-fat milk

1. Steam the fresh spinach in ¼ cup water until wilted, or prepare the frozen spinach according to package directions.
2. Purée the spinach and cooking water in a blender.
3. Melt the margarine in a medium, or 10-inch, skillet, stir in the flour, pepper, and nutmeg, and cook 2 to 3 minutes, stirring often.
4. Add the puréed spinach and cook 5 minutes longer.
5. Just before serving, stir in the yogurt. Thin with low-fat milk to desired consistency.

Yield: 6 servings, 1½ cups
One Serving = 4 tablespoons

Calories: 90
Protein: 5 g
Fat: 4 g
Carbohydrate: 9 g

Fiber: 1.7 g
Cholesterol: 1 mg
Sodium: 150 mg
Potassium: 344 mg

Exchange: 1 vegetable
         ½ low-fat milk

LEMONY SHRIMP CURRY _____

You'll want to prepare this attractive dish for guests. The combination of shrimp with vegetables makes a great presentation. Serve over white or brown rice.

1½ pounds shrimp
¼ cup freshly squeezed lemon juice
⅓ cup cider vinegar
1 teaspoon cumin
1 teaspoon turmeric
¼ to ½ teaspoon cayenne pepper
¼ to ½ teaspoon black pepper
½ teaspoon salt
1 tablespoon vegetable oil
2 tablespoons finely minced ginger root
1 tablespoon finely minced garlic
1 cup finely chopped onion
6 medium tomatoes, seeded and coarsely chopped
2 teaspoons honey
2 teaspoons dark molasses
3 tablespoons finely chopped cilantro
1 to 3 tablespoons green chili pepper, seeded and minced

1. Shell and devein the shrimp, leaving the tail attached. Combine the lemon juice, vinegar, cumin, turmeric, cayenne, black pepper, and ½ teaspoon salt. Add the shrimp and let sit for about 3 minutes.
2. Heat the oil over moderate heat in a large, heavy skillet. Quickly add the ginger, garlic, and onion. Stir-fry for 7 to 8 minutes.
3. Add the marinade from the shrimp and the tomatoes to the skillet and cook for 3 minutes. Add the honey, molasses, and cilantro. Add the shrimp, stir, and sprinkle the green chili on top.
4. Partially cover the skillet and cook over medium heat for 3 to 4 minutes until the shrimp are just pink and firm.

Yield: 6 servings, 6 cups
One Serving = 1 cup

Calories: 158
Protein: 19 g
Fat: 4 g
Carbohydrate: 13 g

Fiber: 2.4 g
Cholesterol: 161 mg
Sodium: 379 mg
Potassium: 571 mg

Exchange: 2 lean meat
　　　　　 2 vegetable

ROULADE OF SOLE _____ EASY, MICROWAVE

½ pound fillet of sole
1 small carrot, cut into fine julienne
½ small zucchini, cut into fine julienne
2 green onions, chopped
1 teaspoon dill weed
1 tablespoon freshly squeezed lemon juice
3 tablespoons dry white wine
Paprika
Lemon wedges

1. Place fish lengthwise on a flat surface. Place carrots, zucchini, and onions crosswise in the center of the fillet.
2. Sprinkle with dill.
3. Roll fish, starting with the narrow, or thin, end, and secure with a toothpick. Place in a microwave-safe dish.
4. Mix lemon juice with wine and pour over the fish roll.
5. Sprinkle with paprika.
6. Loosely cover with plastic wrap and cook in microwave on high for 1 to 2 minutes or until vegetables are tender and fish flakes.
7. Remove to a serving platter and garnish with lemon wedges.

Yield: 2 servings, 8-ounce fish roll
One Serving = 3 ounces

Calories: 118	Fiber: 1.8 g
Protein: 20 g	Cholesterol: 53 mg
Fat: 1 g	Sodium: 99 mg
Carbohydrate: 6 g	Potassium: 513 mg

Exchange: 2 lean meat
          1 vegetable

SHELLFISH AND ARTICHOKE CASSEROLE

½ pound fresh mushrooms, sliced

3 tablespoons margarine

1½ pounds shrimp, shelled, deveined, and cooked (or crabmeat or a
   combination of crabmeat and shrimp)

8 to 10 frozen artichoke hearts, cooked according to package directions,
   coarsely chopped

¼ cup all-purpose flour

1½ cups low-fat milk

½ cup dry sherry

1 tablespoon Worcestershire sauce

⅛ teaspoon salt

Freshly ground black pepper to taste

¼ teaspoon paprika

¼ cup freshly grated Parmesan cheese

1. Preheat oven to 350°F.

2. Sauté mushrooms in a nonstick skillet with 1 teaspoon margarine
until they are soft.

3. In a 3-quart casserole dish, layer mushrooms, shellfish, and artichoke hearts.

4. Melt the remaining margarine in a saucepan. Stir in flour and cook
for 3 minutes.

5. Slowly stir in milk and cook until sauce thickens, stirring often.

6. Add sherry, Worcestershire sauce, salt, pepper, and paprika.

7. Pour sauce over casserole; top with Parmesan cheese.

8. Bake, uncovered, for 30 to 40 minutes until lightly browned.

Yield: 8 servings, 6 cups
One Serving = ¾ cup

Calories: 221
Protein: 22 g
Fat: 7 g
Carbohydrate: 13 g

Fiber: 2 g
Cholesterol: 131 mg
Sodium: 371 mg
Potassium: 540 mg

Exchange: 3 lean meat
          2 vegetable

SHRIMP AND FETA WITH TOFU _____

This version is similar to one in chapter 19. Tofu replaces some of the feta cheese, decreasing calories and fat.

> ¾ **pound medium shrimp, shelled, deveined, and cooked**
> ½ **pound feta cheese, crumbled**
> ½ **pound tofu, drained and crumbled**
> 6 **green onions, finely chopped**
> 4 **teaspoons minced fresh oregano or 1½ teaspoons dried**
> 4 **tomatoes, peeled, cored, seeded, and coarsely chopped**
> **Freshly ground black pepper to taste**
> 1 **pound pasta, cooked**

1. Combine shrimp, feta, tofu, onions, oregano, tomatoes, and pepper in a large bowl. Let mixture stand at room temperature for at least 1 hour.
2. Add warm pasta and toss to coat well.
3. Serve immediately.

Yield: 6 servings, 4½ cups sauce and 6 cups pasta
One Serving = ¾ cup sauce with 1 cup pasta

Calories: 454	Fiber: 3.8 g
Protein: 29 g	Cholesterol: 205 mg
Fat: 14 g	Sodium: 563 mg*
Carbohydrate: 53 g	Potassium: 485 mg

Exchange: 3 starch/bread
               3 medium-fat meat

*High in sodium

SHRIMP WITH CASHEWS

Serve with rice and Pot Stickers (p. 306) for an Oriental dinner.

½ pound small shrimp, shelled and deveined
1 cup yellow onion, finely chopped
1 cup carrots, peeled and shredded
1 cup finely chopped Chinese or regular cabbage
¼ cup finely chopped cashews
2 teaspoons corn oil
1 teaspoon chili oil
1 teaspoon curry powder
½ teaspoon cumin
Freshly ground black pepper to taste

1. In a medium bowl, combine shrimp, onion, carrots, cabbage, and cashews.
2. In a large nonstick pan over medium heat, heat the oils. Add seasonings and sauté 1 minute.
3. Add the shrimp mixture and sauté until heated through, about 5 minutes.
4. Transfer to a serving platter and serve hot. Or refrigerate, covered, and serve cool.

Yield: 4 servings, 3 cups
One Serving = ¾ cup

Calories: 164
Protein: 13 g
Fat: 8 g
Carbohydrate: 11 g

Fiber: 2.5 g
Cholesterol: 85 mg
Sodium: 96 mg
Potassium: 388 mg

Exchange: 2 lean meat
2 vegetable

SNAPPER CREOLE

2 teaspoons margarine
½ teaspoon freshly minced garlic
¼ teaspoon cayenne pepper
½ teaspoon paprika
1 onion, chopped
2 stalks celery, chopped
4 red snapper fillets (approximately 4 to 5 ounces each)
2 tablespoons chopped fresh parsley

1. In a nonstick skillet, melt margarine and stir in garlic, cayenne pepper, and paprika.
2. Add onion and celery and sauté until soft.
3. Add fillets and cook until fish flakes.
4. Remove fish to a serving platter and pour the pan juices over fish; top with parsley and serve.

Yield: 4 servings
One Serving = 1 fillet, 3 ounces

Calories: 164	Fiber: 0.9 g
Protein: 28 g	Cholesterol: 77 mg
Fat: 4 g	Sodium: 160 mg
Carbohydrate: 3 g	Potassium: 511 mg

Exchange: 3 lean meat

TERIYAKI FISH FILLETS ────────────────

Fish cooked in the microwave is moist and flavorful. Your choice of cod, sea bass, halibut, or salmon fillets varies the recipe with unique flavors.

> **2 tablespoons dry sherry**
> **1 tablespoon low-sodium soy sauce**
> **1 tablespoon olive oil**
> **2 to 3 teaspoons freshly grated ginger root**
> **1 teaspoon honey**
> **1 to 2 cloves garlic, minced**
> **1 pound fish fillets, ¾ inch thick**

1. In a shallow dish, combine sherry, soy sauce, oil, ginger root, honey, garlic, and 2 tablespoons water. Mix well. Add fish fillets in a single layer. Marinate at room temperature for 20 minutes or refrigerate for up to 4 hours, turning at least twice.

2. Remove fillets from marinade and transfer marinade to a small saucepan. Place fillets in a single layer in a steamer, cover, and steam for 5 to 8 minutes or until fish is opaque and flakes easily when tested with a fork at the thickest part.

3. Meanwhile, warm marinade and drizzle over fish before serving.

Microwave
Marinate the fish in a microwave-safe dish. Cover dish with a vented plastic wrap and cook in microwave on high for 5 minutes or until fish is opaque and flakes easily when tested with a fork.

Yield: 4 servings
One Serving = 3 ounces

Calories: 156	Fiber: 0.1 g
Protein: 22 g	Cholesterol: 60 mg
Fat: 5 g	Sodium: 244 mg
Carbohydrate: 4 g	Potassium: 332 mg

Exchange: 3 lean meat

16

DESSERTS

DESSERT does have a place in the diabetic diet, but we have modified its definition. Although desserts are often associated with sugar- and fat-laden spectacles, the new dessert is a light end to a well-balanced meal. Natural and more healthful ingredients, such as fruits, fruit juices, spices, and flavorings (vanilla, cinnamon, nutmeg), replace sugars.

The American Diabetes Association has taken a position that allows the use of small amounts of different types of sugars in the diet — contingent upon good blood glucose control. We have used a variety of sweeteners in our recipes, including, in some cases, table sugar (or sucrose) if it does not exceed ¾ teaspoon per serving. We have used some fructose as a sweetener because it has more sweetening power than table sugar — 1 teaspoon of fructose tastes sweeter than 1 teaspoon of sucrose. Also, if diabetes is well controlled, fructose is less likely than sucrose to cause a rise in blood glucose.

Noncaloric sweeteners such as Equal, Sunette, and Sweet 'N Low offer a way to sweeten foods without adding calories and increasing carbohydrate intake. A few of our recipes call for the use of noncaloric sweeteners to achieve a desired level of sweetness, yet keep calorie content and portion sizes within reasonable limits.

In addition to everything else, our dessert recipes are nutritious. We have kept the fat and sugar to a minimum and maximized the nutritional value. Good-tasting desserts should be good for you!

HOW TO IMPROVE DESSERT AND
BAKED GOODS RECIPES

1. If you want to increase the fiber content of a recipe, you can generally substitute one half the amount of all-purpose flour with whole wheat or whole wheat pastry flour.
2. Leavening agents such as baking powder and baking soda contain a great deal of sodium, but you cannot omit or decrease them, or the product will not rise. Look in your supermarket or a specialty store for low-sodium baking products.
3. Fats and oils (including lard, butter, vegetable shortening, cooking oils, margarines, and vegetable fats) add tenderness, crispness, lightness, and volume to a recipe. In general, the amount of fat in a cookie or bread can be cut back by a quarter to a half and still produce an acceptable product. Replace all saturated fats in a recipe with appropriate poly- or monounsaturated fats. Add additional liquid to make up for some of the fat that has been cut from a recipe.
4. Sugar and other sweeteners add flavor, color, tenderness, and crispness. You can usually reduce substantially the sugar content of a recipe, however, without affecting the quality of your product. Flavors that can enhance the sweetness of a recipe without adding calories and simple carbohydrate include vanilla, cinnamon, and nutmeg.
5. Eggs form the network of a baked good along with flour. Eggs also add flavor, color, and moisture. Substitute two egg whites for one whole egg or use egg substitutes to reduce the cholesterol content of a recipe.

Applesauce Cupcakes with
  Creamy Cheese Frosting
Banana "Ice Cream"
Burritos de Manzana
Chocolate Almond Filling
Chocolate Mousse Pie
Cinnamon Raisin Rice
  Pudding
Chocolate Parfaits Pronto
Fall Fruit Compote
Fresh Fruit Kabobs

Cream Puffs
Creamy Berry Filling
Fruit Medley
Harvest Fruit with Yogurt
  Dressing
Tropical Fruit Compote
Pinto Bean Cake
Strawberry Dippers
Strawberry Pie
Low-Calorie Chocolate
  Pudding

APPLESAUCE CUPCAKES _____

Frost with Creamy Cheese Frosting.

⅓ cup margarine
1 egg
2 tablespoons honey
3 tablespoons unsweetened apple juice
1¾ cups sifted all-purpose flour
1 teaspoon baking soda
1 teaspoon cinnamon
1½ teaspoons nutmeg
1 cup unsweetened applesauce
1 teaspoon vanilla
2 tablespoons raisins
Nonstick vegetable spray

1. Preheat oven to 375°F.
2. Cream margarine until fluffy.
3. Beat egg, honey, and apple juice together; add to margarine and blend.
4. Sift together dry ingredients. Add to margarine mixture alternately with applesauce, mixing well after each addition.
5. Stir in vanilla and raisins.
6. Spoon into 12 cupcake pans that have been coated with nonstick vegetable spray. Bake 15 to 20 minutes.

Yield: 12 cupcakes
One Serving = 1 cupcake

Calories: 141	Fiber: 1 g
Protein: 2 g	Cholesterol: 23 mg
Fat: 6 g	Sodium: 184 mg
Carbohydrate: 20 g	Potassium: 60 mg

Exchange: 1 starch/bread
         ½ fruit
         1 fat

CREAMY CHEESE FROSTING

For Applesauce Cupcakes.

1 cup low-fat cottage cheese	½ teaspoon vanilla
3 tablespoons margarine	2 packages Equal
1 tablespoon nonfat milk	2 teaspoons unsweetened cocoa powder

Mix all ingredients in a blender or food processor until smooth.

Yield: 16 servings, 1 cup
One Serving = 1 tablespoon

Calories: 33
Protein: 2 g
Fat: 2 g
Carbohydrate: 1 g

Fiber: trace
Cholesterol: 1 mg
Sodium: 86 mg
Potassium: 20 mg

Exchange: ½ fat

BANANA "ICE CREAM" _____ EASY

This recipe comes courtesy of Mary Donkersloot, R.D., a nutritionist in private practice in San Diego.

4 ripe bananas
1 teaspoon grated orange peel
1 teaspoon vanilla
Fresh mint leaves for garnish

1. Peel, slice, and freeze bananas.
2. Thaw slightly and purée in a blender or food processor.
3. Add vanilla and orange peel and mix.
4. Pour into 4 serving dishes and garnish with mint.

Yield: 4 servings, 2 cups
One Serving = ½ cup

Calories: 106
Protein: 1 g
Fat: <1 g
Carbohydrate: 27 g

Fiber: 2.3 g
Cholesterol: 0
Sodium: 1 mg
Potassium: 452 mg

Exchange: 1½ fruit

BURRITOS DE MANZANA

Serve these Mexican treats topped with low-fat Cheddar cheese, plain yogurt, or a low-calorie whipped topping.

1 tablespoon honey
½ cup unsweetened apple juice
3 cups tart apples, unpeeled and sliced
¼ teaspoon cinnamon
¼ teaspoon nutmeg
1 teaspoon grated lemon peel
½ teaspoon vanilla
1 tablespoon cornstarch
1 tablespoon freshly squeezed lemon juice
5 flour tortillas, 8-inch diameter or smaller
Nonstick vegetable spray
2 teaspoons margarine, melted

1. In a 4- to 6-quart pan, over low heat, dissolve honey in apple juice.
2. Carefully stir in apples, cinnamon, nutmeg, lemon peel, and vanilla. Cook until just tender.
3. Mix cornstarch with lemon juice and add to apples.
4. Raise heat to medium and cook, stirring gently, until liquid boils and thickens and apples are tender, about 2 minutes; remove from heat.
5. If made ahead, cool; then cover and chill.
6. Just before filling the tortillas, warm mixture over low heat until heated through.
7. Wrap flour tortillas in foil; heat in a 350°F oven for about 20 minutes. Place 3 tablespoons of filling down the center of each tortilla. Roll up to enclose filling and place burritos, seam side down, in a 9 × 12-inch baking dish coated with nonstick spray.
8. Bake, uncovered, in a preheated 400°F oven for 20 minutes or until slightly browned.
9. Brush with melted margarine and broil until golden brown, about 3 to 5 minutes.

Yield: 5 servings
One Serving = 1 burrito

Calories: 240
Protein: 4 g
Fat: 6 g
Carbohydrate: 47 g

Fiber: 3.2 g
Cholesterol: 4 mg
Sodium: 215 mg
Potassium: 164 mg

Exchange: 1½ starch/bread
1½ fruit
1 fat

CHOCOLATE ALMOND FILLING ⸺

Use as a filling for Cream Puffs (p. 282).

1 envelope reduced-calorie whipped topping mix
⅓ cup unsweetened cocoa powder
⅓ cup nonfat milk, chilled
3 tablespoons Neufchâtel cheese, softened
½ teaspoon almond extract

1. Combine whipped topping mix and cocoa in a deep, narrow-bottomed bowl; add milk.
2. Using an electric mixer, beat at high speed for 4 minutes or until light and fluffy.
3. Add Neufchâtel cheese, beating until well blended.
4. Stir in almond extract.
5. Spoon into Cream Puff shells.

Yield: 8 servings, about 2 cups
One Serving = ¼ cup filling

Calories: 35
Protein: 2 g
Fat: 2 g
Carbohydrate: 2 g

Fiber: trace
Cholesterol: 5 mg
Sodium: 29 mg
Potassium: 83 mg

Exchange: ½ nonfat milk

CHOCOLATE MOUSSE PIE

10 chocolate or vanilla wafers
1 tablespoon margarine, melted
1 package unflavored gelatin
1½ cups nonfat milk
¾ cup part-skim ricotta cheese
½ cup unsweetened cocoa powder + extra for dusting
10 to 12 packages Equal
1 teaspoon vanilla
1 envelope reduced-calorie whipped topping mix

Crust
1. In a blender or food processor, crush cookie wafers.
2. Mix with melted margarine.
3. Press into an ungreased 9-inch pie plate and freeze for 1 hour.

Filling
1. Sprinkle gelatin over ½ cup of nonfat milk.
2. Let stand for 10 minutes, then heat over low heat until gelatin is dissolved.
3. Blend with ricotta cheese, cocoa powder, Equal, vanilla, and the remaining milk.
4. Pour into pie crust and chill.

Topping
1. Prepare whipped topping according to package directions.
2. Spread over top of chilled pie and dust with cocoa powder. Return to refrigerator and chill.

Yield: 8 servings
One Serving = ⅛ pie

Calories: 116
Protein: 7 g
Fat: 5 g
Carbohydrate: 11 g

Fiber: 0
Cholesterol: 11 mg
Sodium: 86 mg
Potassium: 221 mg

Exchange: 1 low-fat milk

CINNAMON RAISIN RICE PUDDING ———— MICROWAVE

A creamy dessert that is higher in fiber than traditional rice puddings.
Serve with a dollop of low-fat vanilla yogurt.

¾ cup cooked brown rice	¼ teaspoon cinnamon
¾ cup cooked white rice	¼ teaspoon nutmeg
¼ cup raisins	1 cup nonfat milk
¼ cup fructose	1 egg, slightly beaten
1 tablespoon all-purpose flour	1 teaspoon vanilla
⅛ teaspoon pumpkin pie spice	2 tablespoons finely chopped walnuts

1. Preheat oven to 350°F.
2. Combine ingredients and pour into a 1-quart baking dish. Place dish in a shallow baking pan filled 1 inch deep with water.
3. Bake 45 minutes or until center of pudding is firm.
4. Serve cool or warm.

Microwave
1. Combine cooked brown and white rice and raisins in a 1-quart microwave-safe casserole dish and set aside.
2. Combine fructose, flour, and spices in a small, microwave-safe bowl and gradually stir in milk and egg. Cook in microwave on high for 3 minutes or until mixture is bubbly. Be sure to stir after each minute.
3. Add vanilla to liquid mixture; then pour over rice. Mix well to a creamy consistency. Sprinkle with walnuts.
4. Cover dish and cook on medium for 3 to 5 minutes or until center is set.
5. Serve cool or warm.

Yield: 6 servings, 3 cups
One Serving = ½ cup

Calories: 158	Fiber: 2 g
Protein: 4 g	Cholesterol: 46 mg
Fat: 3 g	Sodium: 37 mg
Carbohydrate: 29 g	Potassium: 195 mg

Exchange: 2 starch/bread

CHOCOLATE PARFAITS PRONTO QUICK

    1 envelope reduced-calorie whipped topping mix
    2 tablespoons unsweetened cocoa powder
    ½ cup nonfat milk
    1 teaspoon vanilla

1. In a mixing bowl, combine topping mix and cocoa.
2. Blend in milk and vanilla.
3. Beat on high speed, about 2 minutes. Continue beating until light and fluffy.
4. Spoon ½ cup of the mixture into serving dishes.
5. Chill until serving time.

Yield: 4 servings, 2 cups
One Serving = ½ cup

Calories: 23	Fiber: 0
Protein: 2 g	Cholesterol: <1 mg
Fat: <1 g	Sodium: 18 mg
Carbohydrate: 3 g	Potassium: 97 mg

Exchange: 1 serving = free

FALL FRUIT COMPOTE EASY

This traditional Passover dish is delicious as a sweet side dish at any time of the year. You can easily double the recipe.

    2 small Golden Delicious apples, cored, peeled, and diced
    2 tablespoons dark or golden raisins
    4 dates, pitted and chopped
    ¼ teaspoon cinnamon
    1 package Equal
    1 tablespoon finely chopped walnuts

1. In a small saucepan, combine the apples, raisins, dates, and cinnamon with 1 tablespoon water. Cook over medium heat until apples are softened, about 10 minutes.
2. Transfer to a small glass or stainless steel bowl and stir in Equal and walnuts. (Do not use an aluminum bowl, which may cause color and flavor changes in food.)

3. Cover and refrigerate overnight to allow flavors to blend.

Yield: 4 servings, 2 cups
One Serving = ½ cup

Calories: 86
Protein: 1 g
Fat: 1 g
Carbohydrate: 21 g

Fiber: 2.9 g
Cholesterol: 0
Sodium: 1 mg
Potassium: 179 mg

Exchange: 1½ fruit

FRESH FRUIT KABOBS ⸻ QUICK

1 large apple, quartered
1 banana, peeled and thickly sliced
1 cup strawberries, hulled
1 orange, peeled and sectioned
4 bamboo stick skewers
Cinnamon
Nutmeg

1. Arrange fruits on skewers, alternating colors and varieties.
2. Sprinkle with cinnamon and nutmeg.

Yield: 4 skewers
One Serving = 1 skewer

Calories: 97
Protein: 1 g
Fat: 1 g
Carbohydrate: 23 g

Fiber: 4.5 g
Cholesterol: 0
Sodium: 1 mg
Potassium: 309 mg

Exchange: 1½ fruit

CREAM PUFFS

Fill these puffs with Crab Mornay (p. 113), Chocolate Almond Filling (p. 277), Creamy Berry Filling (p. 283), or one of your own favorites.

> **1 cup nonfat milk**
> **⅓ cup margarine**
> **1 cup flour**
> **⅛ teaspoon salt**
> **8 egg whites, or 1 cup egg substitute, at room temperature**
> **Nonstick vegetable spray**

1. Combine milk and margarine in a saucepan and bring to a boil.
2. Add flour and salt, stirring quickly with a wooden spoon.
3. When the paste begins to look smooth, stir faster.
4. After the paste becomes dry and does not stick to the spoon, remove from heat. Do not overcook or overstir!
5. After 2 minutes, beat in egg whites. The paste has reached its desired consistency when it stands up on the end of the spoon.
6. Spoon small ¾-inch dough balls onto a cookie sheet coated with nonstick spray, smoothing down any rough points.
7. Sprinkle lightly with water.
8. Bake in a preheated 400°F oven for 10 minutes. Reduce heat to 350°F and bake 25 minutes longer. Remove from the oven when firm to the touch. Cool before filling.
9. Slice horizontally with a sharp knife and fill.

Yield: 10 servings, 10 4-inch shells
One Serving = 1 shell

Calories: 117	Fiber: 0 g
Protein: 5 g	Cholesterol: 0 mg
Fat: 6 g	Sodium: 82 mg
Carbohydrate: 10 g	Potassium: 91 mg

Exchange: 1 starch/bread
           1 fat

CREAMY BERRY FILLING ─────────────────────────

Use as a filling for Cream Puffs (p. 282).

⅔ cup frozen raspberries or strawberries, in unsweetened syrup, thawed
½ tablespoon cornstarch
1 envelope reduced-calorie whipped topping mix
½ cup nonfat milk, chilled

1. Drain berries, reserving ⅔ cup of juice. In a small saucepan, combine juice and cornstarch and cook over medium heat, stirring constantly, until mixture comes to a boil.
2. Cook 1 minute, or until thickened, continuing to stir constantly. Remove from heat.
3. Cool slightly and stir in berries. Chill.
4. Combine whipped topping mix and milk in a deep, chilled bowl.
5. Beat at high speed using an electric mixer for 4 minutes or until topping is light and fluffy.
6. Fold chilled berry mixture into whipped topping mixture.
7. Spoon into Cream Puff shells.

Yield: 8 servings, 2 cups
One Serving = 4 tablespoons

Calories: 40
Protein: 1 g
Fat: <1 g
Carbohydrate: 8 g

Fiber: 1.2 g
Cholesterol: <1 mg
Sodium: 12 mg
Potassium: 64 mg

Exchange: 1 serving = 1 fruit

FRUIT MEDLEY _____ QUICK

1 package unflavored gelatin
1 cup unsweetened applesauce
½ cup crushed pineapple in its own juice, drained
½ cup blueberries or hulled strawberries
1 small banana, peeled and sliced
8 ounces plain nonfat yogurt
Vanilla

1. Combine gelatin and applesauce in a saucepan.
2. Heat to dissolve gelatin over medium heat.
3. Remove from heat and stir in remaining ingredients.
4. Spoon into 6 serving dishes and chill until set.

Yield: 6 servings, 3 cups
One Serving = ½ cup

Calculated with strawberries:

Calories: 71
Protein: 4 g
Fat: <1 g
Carbohydrate: 14 g

Fiber: 1.6 g
Cholesterol: 0.7 mg
Sodium: 32 mg
Potassium: 267 mg

Exchange: 1 fruit

HARVEST FRUIT WITH YOGURT DRESSING _____ EASY

1 cup cored and cubed red apple
1 cup halved red seedless grapes
1 cup banana slices
1 cup cored and cubed pear

Dressing
8 ounces vanilla low-fat yogurt
½ cup evaporated skim milk
1 tablespoon honey

¼ cup chopped almonds
Cinnamon

1. Combine fruits in a medium bowl. Spoon ½ cup mixture into each of 8 serving dishes.
2. In a small bowl, combine yogurt, milk, and honey. Drizzle dressing over fruit.
3. Sprinkle with almonds and cinnamon.

Yield: 8 servings, 4 cups
One Serving = ½ cup fruit, 1½ ounces dressing

Calories: 131	Fiber: 2.5 g
Protein: 4 g	Cholesterol: 2 mg
Fat: 3 g	Sodium: 38 mg
Carbohydrate: 24 g	Potassium: 338 mg

Exchange: 1 fruit
          ½ low-fat milk

TROPICAL FRUIT COMPOTE

1 banana, peeled and sliced

1 cup unsweetened pineapple chunks, drained

1 kiwi fruit, peeled and sliced

¼ honeydew melon or cantaloupe, diced (about ½ cup)

2 teaspoons grated orange peel

¼ teaspoon nutmeg

1 tablespoon chopped macadamia nuts

1. Preheat oven to 400°F.
2. Arrange fruits in a baking dish.
3. Sprinkle with orange peel, nutmeg, and nuts.
4. Bake for 10 to 15 minutes, or until hot. Serve warm.

Yield: 4 servings, 2 cups
One Serving = ½ cup

Calories: 82	Fiber: 2.3 g
Protein: 1 g	Cholesterol: 0 mg
Fat: 2 g	Sodium: 64 mg
Carbohydrate: 17 g	Potassium: 322 mg

Exchange: 1½ fruit

PINTO BEAN CAKE

This is a dense, moist cake with a surprisingly good taste. Because it is an exception to our low-fat guidelines, include it only on special occasions.

¼ cup fructose
½ cup margarine, softened
2 eggs
2 cups pinto beans, cooked and
    mashed
1 cup all-purpose flour
1 teaspoon baking soda

1 teaspoon cinnamon
½ teaspoon ground cloves
½ teaspoon allspice
2 cups diced apples
¾ cup raisins
¼ cup chopped walnuts
2 teaspoons vanilla

1. With an electric mixer or food processor, cream fructose and margarine until smooth. Stir in eggs and beans.
2. Sift all dry ingredients together and add to sugar mixture.
3. Add apples, raisins, nuts, and vanilla.
4. Pour into a lightly oiled 10-inch angel food cake or bundt pan and bake in a preheated 375°F oven for 45 minutes or until done.

Yield: 12 servings
One Serving = ¹⁄₁₂ cake

Calories: 210
Protein: 6 g
Fat: 10 g
Carbohydrate: 25 g

Fiber: 2.5 g
Cholesterol: 46 mg
Sodium: 113 mg
Potassium: 60 mg

Exchange: 1½ starch/bread
            2 fat

STRAWBERRY DIPPERS ———————————— QUICK

This recipe comes compliments of Mary Donkersloot, R.D., a nutrition consultant in San Diego.

1 teaspoon part-skim ricotta cheese
½ cup plain nonfat yogurt
2 packages Equal
2½ cups strawberries (with long stems, if possible)

1. Combine ricotta cheese, yogurt, and Equal; mix thoroughly.
2. Dip strawberries into mixture and serve.

Yield: 2 servings, ⅔ cup yogurt mixture and 2½ cups strawberries
One Serving = ⅓ cup mixture and 1¼ cups strawberries

Calories: 66
Protein: 4 g
Fat: <1 g
Carbohydrate: 12 g

Fiber: 2.5 g
Cholesterol: 2 mg
Sodium: 37 mg
Potassium: 301 mg

Exchange: 1 fruit

STRAWBERRY PIE

1 cup crushed chocolate wafers
1 teaspoon margarine, melted
1 cup plain low-fat yogurt
1 cup part-skim ricotta cheese
2 teaspoons sugar

1 teaspoon vanilla
1 package unflavored gelatin
1 cup sliced strawberries
Additional strawberries for
    garnish

1. Combine chocolate wafer crumbs with margarine; press into a 9-inch pie pan and freeze for 1 hour.
2. Mix yogurt, ricotta cheese, sugar, and vanilla in a blender or food processor.
3. Dissolve gelatin in 1 tablespoon of cold water. Stir in 3 tablespoons of boiling water.
4. Add gelatin mixture to blender or food processor and mix well.
5. Arrange sliced strawberries in pie crust. Pour yogurt mixture evenly over the top.
6. Chill several hours until firm.
7. Garnish top with more sliced strawberries.

Yield: 12 servings
One Serving = 1/12 pie

Calories: 117
Protein: 5 g
Fat: 4 g
Carbohydrate: 14 g

Fiber: 0.3 g
Cholesterol: 16 mg
Sodium: 105 mg
Potassium: 107 mg

Exchange: 1 starch/bread
          1 fat

LOW-CALORIE CHOCOLATE PUDDING _____

A cooked, custardy pudding, very creamy and delicious.

1 quart low-fat milk (4 cups)	**2 teaspoons sugar**
¼ cup cornstarch	**2 eggs**
½ teaspoon salt	**6 packages Equal**
¼ cup unsweetened cocoa powder	**1 tablespoon vanilla**

1. In a nonstick pan, scald 3½ cups milk, heating only until bubbles appear around the edge.
2. Combine the remaining ½ cup milk with cornstarch, salt, and cocoa; stir into hot milk.
3. Add sugar and stir over very low heat until mixture thickens.
4. In a large mixing bowl, beat eggs and slowly beat some of the hot milk mixture into the eggs. (Beat continuously to prevent eggs from curdling.)
5. Return egg mixture to the saucepan and cook over very low heat, stirring constantly, until pudding is smooth and thick. Do not allow to boil.
6. When thick, remove from heat and stir in Equal and vanilla.
7. Pour into a bowl or 8 dessert dishes and chill thoroughly.

Yield: 8 servings, 4 cups
One Serving = ½ cup

Calories: 118	Fiber: 1.2 g
Protein: 6 g	Cholesterol: 78 mg
Fat: 5 g	Sodium: 212 mg
Carbohydrate: 14 g	Potassium: 259 mg

Exchange: 1 low-fat milk

17

THIS AND THAT

THESE RECIPES offer healthful alternatives to high-fat, high-calorie, high-cholesterol foods. Don't feel deprived of sour cream, syrup, cake frosting, or whipped topping — try our recipes and enjoy the tasty results!

Fruit Syrup
Chicken Stock
Savory Seasonings
Herb Croutons
Homemade Egg Substitute
Marinara Sauce

Sour Cream Substitute
Spicy Catsup
Tartar Sauce
Tofu Spread
Whipped Topping

FRUIT SYRUP ———————————————— QUICK

Use as a topping on waffles or pancakes.

1 tablespoon reduced-sugar jelly or jam
2 to 3 teaspoons warm water

Mix jelly with water. Add water slowly to obtain desired consistency.

Yield: 3 servings, 2 to 3 tablespoons syrup
One Serving = 1 tablespoon

Calories: 15
Protein: <1 g
Fat: 0
Carbohydrate: 4 g

Fiber: 0 g
Cholesterol: 0
Sodium: 0
Potassium: 9 mg

Exchange: 1 serving = free

CHICKEN STOCK

1 4-pound chicken, including neck and giblets (except liver)
12½ cups water
1 large onion pierced with 2 cloves
2 leeks, halved lengthwise
2 carrots
1 stalk celery, halved
1 teaspoon salt
A cheesecloth bag filled with the following:
    4 fresh cilantro or parsley sprigs
    ½ teaspoon thyme
    1 clove garlic, unpeeled
    1 large bay leaf

1. Chop the neck and giblets and combine them with the chicken and 12 cups water. Bring the water to a boil, skimming the froth.
2. Add ½ cup water and reduce the heat to a simmer, skimming the froth. Add the onion, leeks, carrots, celery, salt, and cheesecloth bag, and simmer the mixture, continuing to skim the froth, for 2 hours.
3. Remove the chicken from the kettle. Remove the meat and skin from the carcass and reserve the meat for another use.
4. Chop the carcass and return it to the kettle. Simmer the stock, adding boiling water to barely cover the ingredients if necessary, for 2 hours or more.
5. Strain the stock through a fine sieve into a bowl, pressing hard on the solids, and let it cool. Chill the stock and remove the fat. Freeze the stock if desired for later use.

Yield: 12 cups
One Serving = 1 cup

Calories: 39	Fiber: 0
Protein: 5 g	Cholesterol: 0
Fat: 1 g	Sodium: 192 mg
Carbohydrate: <1 g	Potassium: 210 mg

Exchange: ½ lean meat

SAVORY SEASONINGS

Mixing seasonings in parts provides flexibility for quantities. One example for making a small amount is to allow 1 part to equal 1 teaspoon and ½ part to equal ½ teaspoon.

Vegetable/Meat and Poultry
>   1 part marjoram
>   ½ part thyme
>   1 part sweet basil
>   ½ part sage
>   1 part parsley

Italian Herb (for salads, sauces)
>   Equal parts:
>   oregano
>   sweet basil
>   rosemary
>   sage
>   marjoram

Cajun Spice (for spicy dishes)
>   1 part paprika
>   1 part turmeric
>   ½ part cayenne pepper
>   1 part cumin
>   ¼ part black pepper

Chinese Five-Spice (for Oriental dishes)
>   Equal parts:
>   anise
>   fennel
>   white pepper
>   cloves
>   cinnamon

Exchange: Free

HERB CROUTONS _____ QUICK

Transform stale bread into homemade croutons. Sprinkle onto salads or soups.

4 slices stale whole wheat bread
Suggested seasonings:
    garlic powder
    onion powder
    basil
    oregano
    Butter Buds

1. Cut bread into small cubes and place on a nonstick cookie sheet.
2. Sprinkle bread cubes lightly with water and with a combination of the suggested seasonings to taste.
3. Bake in a preheated 250°F oven about 10 to 15 minutes or until bread cubes are crunchy.

Yield: 6 servings, about 1½ cups
One Serving = ¼ cup

Calories: 41	Fiber: 2 g
Protein: 2 g	Cholesterol: 0
Fat: <1 g	Sodium: 106 mg
Carbohydrate: 8 g	Potassium: 32 mg

Exchange: ½ starch/bread

HOMEMADE EGG SUBSTITUTE _____ QUICK

You can use this recipe in place of a commercial egg substitute. It is considerably cheaper!

6 egg whites
¼ cup nonfat dry milk
1 tablespoon vegetable oil

1. Combine all ingredients in a mixing bowl and blend until smooth.
2. Store in a jar in the refrigerator up to 1 week. (This mixture also freezes well.)

To prepare scrambled eggs: fry slowly over low heat in a nonstick frying pan.

Yield: 4 servings, 1 cup
One Serving = ¼ cup (1 egg equivalent)

Calories: 69
Protein: 7 g
Fat: 3 g
Carbohydrate: 3 g

Fiber: 0
Cholesterol: <1 mg
Sodium: 98 mg
Potassium: 140 mg

Exchange: 1 lean meat

MARINARA SAUCE ————————————————— EASY

A simple sauce to serve over your favorite pasta.

¼ onion, chopped
2 to 3 cloves garlic, minced
1 teaspoon vegetable oil
1 can (28 ounces) plum tomatoes, chopped
1 teaspoon basil
1 teaspoon oregano

1. In a medium saucepan, sauté onion and garlic in oil until soft.
2. Add tomatoes and herbs and bring to a boil.
3. Simmer for at least 20 minutes or as long as a few hours, until desired consistency is obtained.

Yield: 5 to 7 servings, 2½ to 3½ cups
One Serving = ½ cup

Calories: 30
Protein: 1 g
Fat: 1 g
Carbohydrate: 5 g

Fiber: 1.8 g
Cholesterol: 0
Sodium: 9 mg
Potassium: 235 mg

Exchange: 1 vegetable

SOUR CREAM SUBSTITUTE

This recipe makes a great dip for crackers, pretzels, bread sticks, fresh vegetables, or berries; a dressing for fruit or vegetable salads; a topping for potatoes, cooked vegetables, and tortillas; or a spread for bagels. Use it in any recipe that does not require heating. (In recipes that do require heating, plain nonfat yogurt is a good sour cream substitute.)

1 cup low-fat cottage cheese
2 tablespoons buttermilk or nonfat milk
2 teaspoons freshly squeezed lemon juice

Blend cottage cheese, milk, and lemon juice in a blender or with a mixer until smooth. Scrape the sides of the container often with a rubber spatula while blending.

Yield: 8 servings, 1 cup
One Serving = 2 tablespoons

Calories: 28
Protein: 4 g
Fat: <1 g
Carbohydrate: 2 g

Fiber: 0
Cholesterol: 2 mg
Sodium: 116 mg
Potassium: 36 mg

Exchange: ½ lean meat

SPICY CATSUP

1 tablespoon sugar
½ tablespoon white wine vinegar
1 can (6 ounces) tomato paste
2 teaspoons Worcestershire sauce
Dash of Tabasco sauce
2 to 3 cloves garlic, pressed or minced
Freshly ground black pepper to taste
½ cup water

1. In a bowl, dissolve sugar in vinegar; add remaining ingredients, except water, and mix well.
2. Add water to desired consistency.
3. Refrigerate until ready to use.

Yield: 16 servings, 1 cup
One Serving = 1 tablespoon

Calories: 14
Protein: <1 g
Fat: <1 g
Carbohydrate: 3 g

Fiber: 0
Cholesterol: 0
Sodium: 7 mg
Potassium: 103 mg

Exchange: Free

TARTAR SAUCE ———————————————— EASY

This sauce is especially good with Fish Tacos (p. 262)! Or serve it with your favorite fish recipe.

¼ cup reduced-calorie mayonnaise
2 teaspoons pickle relish
½ teaspoon mustard
½ tablespoon freshly squeezed lemon juice
½ tablespoon white vinegar

Combine all ingredients. Chill.

Yield: 4 servings, ¼ cup
One Serving = 1 tablespoon

Calories: 54
Protein: <1 g
Fat: 5 g
Carbohydrate: 2 g

Fiber: trace
Cholesterol: 10 mg
Sodium: 149 mg
Potassium: 4 mg

Exchange: 1 fat

TOFU SPREAD _____ QUICK

Serve on whole wheat bread with tomato and alfalfa sprouts for a unique sandwich.

1 pound tofu
1 tablespoon Dijon-style mustard
½ tablespoon curry powder
1 tablespoon reduced-calorie mayonnaise
¼ cup chopped green onion
Freshly ground black pepper to taste

1. Drain tofu and mash with a fork until crumbled.
2. Add other ingredients and mix until creamy.

Yield: 6 servings, 3 cups
One Serving = ½ cup

Calories: 70		Fiber: 0.1 g	
Protein: 6 g		Cholesterol: 2 mg	
Fat: 4 g		Sodium: 60 mg	
Carbohydrate: 3 g		Potassium: 54 mg	

Exchange: 1 medium-fat meat

WHIPPED TOPPING

Combine with fresh fruit for a parfait dessert or serve over Pinto Bean Cake (p. 286). Add 3 or 4 packets of sugar substitute for a *sweetened* dessert whipped topping.

1 teaspoon unflavored gelatin	**½ cup ice water**
2 teaspoons cold water	**½ cup nonfat milk**
3 tablespoons boiling water	**3 tablespoons vegetable oil**

1. Soften gelatin with cold water. Add the boiling water and stir until gelatin is completely dissolved. Cool to room temperature.
2. Pour ice water and milk into a chilled mixing bowl. Beat at high speed until the mixture forms stiff peaks.
3. Add oil and gelatin, continuing to beat until mixed.
4. Place in freezer for 10 to 15 minutes. Then transfer to refrigerator.
5. Stir before using.

Yield: 24 servings, 1½ cups
One Serving = 1 tablespoon

Calories: 17	Fiber: 0
Protein: <1 g	Cholesterol: 0.1 mg
Fat: 1.7 g	Sodium: 3 mg
Carbohydrate: <1 g	Potassium: 8 mg

Exchange: Free

18

SNACKS
FOR KIDS

SNACK FOODS in this section are for the child who must monitor sugar intake but needs calories for growth. These are recipes that kids can help create and are easy to pack for snacks. Substitute Lettuce Rolls for a change from luncheon sand-wiches and try stuffing them with your child's favorite fill-ing. Cereal Crunch and Apple Snacks are quick and tasty after-school ideas. Banana Smoothies (p. 100), Spiced Co-coa (p. 102), and Bean Dip with No-Fry Tortilla Chips (p. 111) are other good snacks for children. Your child will have no problem avoiding sugary or salty snacks if he or she has a supply of good-tasting snack alternatives.

Cereal Crunch   Lettuce Rolls
Apple Snacks   Mini Pizza Bread Snack
Chocolate Banana Pudding

Quick snacks:

Food	Amount	Grams Carbohydrate	Calories
Low-fat milk	8 ounces	11.7	121
Animal crackers	8 crackers	16.8	90
Graham crackers	3 2 × 2-inch squares	15.4	81
String cheese sticks (skim milk)	1 ounce	0.8	72
Sugar-free pudding	½ cup	13.0	90
Rice or popcorn cakes	2 rounds	16.0	80

Food	Amount	Grams Carbohydrate	Calories
Bread sticks	2 4½-inch sticks	15.1	77
Apple Oatmeal Muffin*	1 muffin	17.0	105
Nonfat yogurt with berries	1½ cups	22.0	170
Banana "Ice Cream"*	½ cup	27.0	106

*See index for recipes.

Snacks containing a significant amount of glucose, good for low blood sugars:

Food	Amount	Grams Carbohydrate	Calories
Raisins	2 tablespoons	14.2	54
Apple juice	½ cup	14.5	58
Orange juice	½ cup	12.8	54
Grape juice	⅓ cup	12.6	51

CEREAL CRUNCH ———————————————— QUICK

1 cup unsalted pretzel twists
1½ cups Cheerios
1½ cups Crispix cereal
⅓ cup raisins
¼ cup unsalted dry-roasted peanuts

1. Mix all ingredients in a large bowl.
2. Serve as a snack mix.

Yield: 4 servings, approximately 4 cups
One Serving = 1 cup

Calories: 213
Protein: 5 g
Fat: 5 g
Carbohydrate: 40 g

Fiber: 3.3 g
Cholesterol: 0
Sodium: 206 mg
Potassium: 266 mg

Exchange: 2 starch/bread
 ½ fruit
 1 fat

APPLE SNACKS _____ QUICK

6 tablespoons peanut butter
1 teaspoon honey
3 small apples, cored (mixture of red and green varieties)

1. Mix peanut butter and honey until smooth.
2. Push 2 tablespoons mixture into the center of an apple, making sure to fill it solidly.
3. Wrap apples with plastic wrap and refrigerate for 30 minutes to set the mixture.
4. Remove wrap from apples and slice vertically.

Yield: 3 apples
One Serving = 1 apple with 2 tablespoons peanut butter mixture

Calories: 260
Protein: 8 g
Fat: 15 g
Carbohydrate: 33 g

Fiber: 2.1 g
Cholesterol: 0
Sodium: 37 mg
Potassium: 408 mg

Exchange: 1 high-fat meat
2 fruit
1 fat

CHOCOLATE BANANA PUDDING _____ QUICK

These unique flavors blend together in this easy recipe.

1 medium banana, peeled and sliced
2 cups low-calorie chocolate pudding prepared with 2 cups nonfat milk
2 tablespoons chopped walnuts

1. Divide bananas among 4 small dessert dishes.
2. Top each with ½ cup pudding.
3. Sprinkle with nuts.

Yield: 4 servings, 2 cups
One Serving = ½ cup pudding

Calories: 80
Protein: 5 g
Fat: <1 g
Carbohydrate: 15 g

Fiber: 0.3
Cholesterol: 2 mg
Sodium: 126 mg
Potassium: 316 mg

Exchange: ½ nonfat milk
            ½ fruit

LETTUCE ROLLS —————————————————— QUICK

Substitute for sandwiches in your child's school lunch. Try adding some diced vegetables.

1 tablespoon low-fat cream cheese
1 lettuce leaf (Bibb or red-leaf)
½ teaspoon unsalted sunflower seeds

1. Spread cream cheese on lettuce, being careful not to tear the leaf.
2. Sprinkle sunflower seeds onto cream cheese.
3. Roll lettuce.

Yield: 1 leaf
One Serving = 1 leaf

Calories: 47
Protein: 2 g
Fat: 4 g
Carbohydrate: 1 g

Fiber: 0.2 g
Cholesterol: 11 mg
Sodium: 59 mg
Potassium: 42 mg

Exchange: 1 fat

MINI PIZZA BREAD SNACK ─────────────────── EASY

An easy after-school snack that children can prepare themselves.

1 French bread baguette (12 inches)
1 cup tomato sauce or Marinara Sauce (p. 293)
½ cup freshly grated part-skim mozzarella cheese

1. Slice baguette into 2-inch rounds.
2. Pour tomato sauce into a shallow pan and allow bread to soak in the sauce for a few minutes. Turn bread to absorb sauce on other side.
3. Sprinkle tops with cheese.
4. Place in a toaster oven and cook until cheese is melted and bread is crispy.

Yield: 3 servings, 6 slices
One Serving = 2 slices

Calories: 160
Protein: 12 g
Fat: 7 g
Carbohydrate: 13 g

Fiber: 0.2 g
Cholesterol: 23 mg
Sodium: 747 mg*
Potassium: 347 mg

Exchange: 1 starch/bread
     1 medium-fat meat

*High in sodium

19

CELEBRATIONS AND SPECIAL OCCASIONS (WITH WINE SELECTIONS)

SPECIAL OCCASIONS and celebrations require special foods. Planning a menu for a cocktail party with hors d'oeuvres, a birthday or anniversary dinner, or a luncheon honoring a special friend creates a challenge. This section provides you with the menu ideas and recipes you need to entertain a group of friends healthfully.

Many of the recipes in this section are slightly higher in fat, salt, simple sugar, and calories than what we recommend on a daily basis. However, they feature the use of poly- and monounsaturated fats and are still highly nutritious meals. Remember, plan ahead for one of these "bigger" meals by eating lighter (fewer calories, less salt and fat) earlier in the day. And adjust your medication and activity level accordingly, with the help of your physician.

Some people choose to celebrate a special occasion with an alcoholic drink. For most people whose diabetes is in good control with diet, medication, and exercise, an occasional drink should not be harmful. (See chapter 4 for guidelines.) Alcohol by itself does not raise blood glucose because the body treats it like a fat. But the carbohydrate in beer, wine, liqueurs, and sugary mixers may cause your blood sugar to go up. Therefore, if you choose to imbibe, one of the best types of drinks to choose is wine that is on the dry side. We have asked a well-known master sommelier, Evan Goldstein, coproprietor of Square One restaurant in San Francisco, to make some suggestions for appropriate wines to accompany the entrees from our menus. (Thank you, Evan, for your valuable advice!) But remember, to prevent hypoglycemia, have your drink shortly before eating and do not drink on an empty stomach or omit food from your meal plan — and, most important, *don't overindulge!**

You'll find that these recipes are a little more work to prepare, but highly worthwhile for that occasional special event.

ORIENTAL PARTY OPENERS

Pot Stickers
Party Sushi Rolls
Beef Teriyaki
Shrimp Teriyaki

Recommended wine:

- a dry sake (Japanese wine)

POT STICKERS

Credit for this recipe goes to Mary Donkersloot, R.D., director of Personal Nutrition Management in San Diego.

½ pound ground turkey
1 cup minced cabbage
2 green onions, minced
1 egg or 2 egg whites
1 tablespoon soy sauce
½ teaspoon grated orange peel
½ teaspoon chili oil (optional)
Cornstarch
40 wonton skins, 2 × 2-inch squares, cut into largest circle possible
4 teaspoons vegetable oil
1 cup water

1. Combine turkey, cabbage, onion, egg, soy sauce, orange peel, and chili oil (if desired) in a large bowl and mix well.
2. Dust a plate or cutting board with cornstarch. Set a rounded teaspoon of filling in center of a wonton skin, pressing lightly so filling

*These recommendations should not be used to encourage alcohol consumption by people with diabetes who risk alcohol abuse.

forms a narrow band across the middle. Moisten the rim of skin with water. Bring opposite sides together to form a semicircle. Pinch corners together. Make 3 or 4 pleats along the edge to seal. Transfer pot sticker to the prepared plate or cutting board. Cover with a dry kitchen towel. Repeat with remaining wonton skins and filling.

3. Place 2 heavy 12-inch nonstick skillets over low heat. Add 2 teaspoons vegetable oil to each. Arrange pot stickers in rows, fitting closely together. Increase heat to medium-high and cook until bottoms are deeply golden, about 2 minutes. Watch carefully to prevent burning.

4. Add ½ cup water to each pan and cover immediately. Let steam until skins are translucent, about 3 minutes. Drain and transfer with a slotted spoon to serving dish. Serve immediately with rice vinegar or soy sauce. (You can assemble pot stickers ahead of time and freeze them.)

Yield: 20 servings, 40 pot stickers
One Serving = 2 pot stickers

Calories: 160	Fiber: 1 g
Protein: 6 g	Cholesterol: 44 mg
Fat: 8 g	Sodium: 68 mg
Carbohydrate: 16 g	Potassium: 64 mg

Exchange: 1 starch/bread
        2 fat

PARTY SUSHI ROLLS

Sushi, a representative food of Japan, is a vinegared rice garnished with an assortment of fresh vegetables, fish, and seasonings. You'll find many of the ingredients — and the bamboo mat — at an Oriental food store.

Rice

> 2 cups white, short-grain rice, preferably Japanese
> 3 cups water (or according to rice package directions)
> 3½ tablespoons rice vinegar or white vinegar
> 1 tablespoon sugar
> 1½ teaspoons salt

1. Cook rice in water for about 25 minutes or until all the liquid is absorbed. Spread rice evenly over bottom of a large glass or wooden bowl.
2. Mix vinegar, sugar, and salt together in a small bowl.
3. Sprinkle vinegar mixture generously over the rice. You may not need all of the vinegar mixture. The rice should remain somewhat dry.
4. With a large wooden spoon, mix rice with a slicing motion.
5. Leave the rice in the bowl, covered with a damp cloth.

Rolls

> 1 package large or medium nori seaweed. (Quality nori seaweed must be crisp. Look for a well-sealed package.)
> 1 medium or large bamboo mat for rolling sushi

Fillings
Choose from these combinations:

> 1 cucumber, cut into thin strips the same length as seaweed
> 1 avocado, peeled, pitted, and cut into thin strips
> Fresh cilantro, minced
>
> 2 ounces daikon radish, cut into strips
> 2 ounces pickled ginger
> 4 ounces small shrimp, cooked
>
> 4 ounces prosciutto
> 1 cucumber, cut into thin strips
> 1 avocado, peeled, pitted, and cut into thin strips
> 2 ounces pickled ginger

To Assemble Sushi Rolls

1. Place one sheet of nori seaweed on the bamboo mat.

2. Spread approximately ¾ cup rice onto seaweed; flatten with the back of a spoon. Leave uncovered ⅜ inch (1 cm) at front of sheet and ¾ inch (2 cm) at end of sheet.

3. Place all filling ingredients at center.

4. To form roll, lift one end of the mat and begin to roll and compress the seaweed. Use the mat only to help form the roll. (It may be difficult at first to keep the mat from rolling with the seaweed.)

5. Moisten end of seaweed with a small amount of water to seal the roll.

6. Cut into rounds approximately ½ inch thick.

Yield: 10 servings; 5 rolls, 6 pieces/roll
One Serving = 3 pieces

	With cilantro filling	With shrimp filling	With prosciutto filling
Calories:	79	68	95
Protein:	2 g	3 g	4 g
Fat:	2 g	<1 g	3 g
Carbohydrate:	14 g	13 g	14 g
Fiber:	1.5 g	0.9 g	1.5 g
Cholesterol:	0	13 mg	4 mg
Sodium:	203 mg	215 mg	317 mg
Potassium:	160 mg	100 mg	257 mg
Exchange:	1 starch/bread	1 starch/bread	1 starch/bread ½ fat

BEEF TERIYAKI

2 pounds flank steak (about 2 large steaks)
1 cup dry white wine
½ cup low-sodium soy sauce
2 tablespoons minced onion
1 clove garlic, minced
1 tablespoon freshly squeezed lemon juice
2 tablespoons honey
1 can (10½ ounces) unsalted beef broth or 1 cup homemade
1 teaspoon minced or grated ginger root

1. Slice steaks diagonally across the grain into ½ × 1-inch strips and place in a shallow pan or large bowl.
2. Mix remaining ingredients and pour over meat. Let marinate 1 to 2 hours, turning 3 or 4 times.
3. Thread strips on skewers and grill until meat reaches desired degree of doneness.

Yield: 12 servings
One Serving = 2 ounces

Calories: 110	Fiber: trace
Protein: 13 g	Cholesterol: 38 mg
Fat: 5 g	Sodium: 229 mg
Carbohydrate: 0	Potassium: 197 mg

Exchange: 2 lean meat

SHRIMP TERIYAKI _____

½ cup low-sodium soy sauce
½ cup olive oil
½ cup sherry
1 tablespoon freshly squeezed lemon juice or white vinegar
1 clove garlic, minced
½ teaspoon minced ginger root
1 teaspoon fresh rosemary or ¼ teaspoon dried
1 teaspoon fresh thyme or ¼ teaspoon dried
1 teaspoon fresh oregano or ¼ teaspoon dried
1 teaspoon fresh marjoram or ¼ teaspoon dried
2 pounds large shrimp, shelled and deveined

1. Mix soy sauce, oil, sherry, lemon juice, garlic, ginger root, and herbs together. Pour over shrimp.
2. Let shrimp stand in marinade for approximately 1 hour. Remove shrimp from marinade and broil or grill for 5 to 7 minutes.

Yield: 16 servings
One Serving = 2 shrimp (approximately 1 ounce each)

Calories: 95
Protein: 11 g
Fat: 5 g
Carbohydrate: 1 g

Fiber: trace
Cholesterol: 85 mg
Sodium: 320 mg
Potassium: 144 mg

Exchange: 1 lean meat
          1 fat

AUTUMN FLAVORS

Polenta Appetizer Squares
Lamb and Squash Curry
Basmati brown rice
Salad greens with fresh herbs
Apple Pie Sweetened with Raisins and Dates

Recommended wine:

- a hearty, rich, red wine, such as a Zinfandel, a Rhone red wine from France, a Piemontese red wine from Italy

POLENTA APPETIZER SQUARES

Crust

7 cups water	**1 cup cornmeal, finely ground**
½ teaspoon salt	**¼ teaspoon Italian seasoning**
1 cup cornmeal, stone-ground or coarse	

1. Prepare the polenta by bringing the water and salt to a boil. Slowly add the cornmeal in a thin, steady stream, whisking constantly. Cook, stirring occasionally, for 20 minutes, until the polenta is stiff and leaves the sides of the pan. Spread in a 9 × 13-inch baking dish to a depth of 1½ to 2 inches.
2. Cut the polenta into 30 squares, approximately 2 × 2 inches each. Keep warm in a 250°F oven while you prepare the toppings.

Tomato-Basil Topping

- **3 cups tomatoes, peeled, seeded, and chopped**
- **¼ cup minced fresh basil leaves**
- **4 cloves garlic, crushed**
- **2 tablespoons olive oil**

Sauté the tomatoes, basil, and garlic in olive oil for approximately 5 minutes. Distribute evenly over polenta squares. Bake in the pan for 15 to 20 minutes in a preheated 375°F oven and serve warm.

Sun-Dried Tomato Topping

    2 cups freshly grated part-skim mozzarella cheese
    ½ cup minced sun-dried tomatoes

Combine grated cheese with sun-dried tomatoes and distribute evenly over polenta. Place under broiler for 1 minute.

Chicken, Olive, and Pepper Topping

    2 cups shredded cooked chicken breast (skin removed before cooking)
    1 cup pitted and sliced black olives
    2 cups freshly grated part-skim mozzarella cheese
    ½ cup diced roasted peppers

Layer chicken, olives, cheese, and peppers on top of the polenta squares. Bake in the pan for 15 to 20 minutes in a preheated 375°F oven and serve warm.

Yield: 30 polenta squares
One Serving = 2 polenta squares

	Polenta with Tomato-Basil Topping	*Polenta with Sun-Dried To- mato Topping*	*Polenta with Chicken, Olive, and Pepper Topping*
Calories:	94	112	150
Protein:	2 g	6 g	11 g
Fat:	2 g	3 g	4 g
Carbohydrate:	17 g	15 g	16 g
Fiber:	2.2 g	1.6 g	1.7 g
Cholesterol:	0	8 mg	22 mg
Sodium:	94 mg	172 mg	262 mg
Potassium:	138 mg	62 mg	96 mg
Exchange:	1 starch/bread	1 starch/bread ½ medium- fat meat	1 starch/bread 1½ lean meat

LAMB AND SQUASH CURRY

Serve this delicious stew over steamed white rice or basmati rice for a truly unique flavor

3 onions, chopped
3 cloves garlic, minced
3 tablespoons vegetable oil
¼ cup loosely packed, peeled and minced ginger root
2 tablespoons curry powder
¼ teaspoon red pepper flakes
¼ teaspoon freshly ground black pepper
2 pounds boneless lean lamb shoulder, cut into ½-inch cubes
2½ to 3 pounds butternut squash or pumpkin, peeled, seeded, and cut into ½-inch cubes
1 2-inch piece of cinnamon stick, broken into pieces
1 teaspoon salt
½ cup unsalted homemade or canned beef broth

1. In a kettle, cook the onions and garlic in the oil over moderate heat, stirring occasionally, for 5 to 7 minutes, or until lightly browned.

2. Add the ginger root, curry powder, red pepper flakes, and black pepper, and cook the mixture over moderately low heat, stirring, for 3 minutes.

3. Cover the onion mixture with a layer of the lamb and then a layer of the squash. Push cinnamon stick pieces into the mixture and sprinkle with salt.

4. Pour broth over all and simmer for 1½ hours or until lamb and squash are tender.

5. Add salt and pepper to taste. Stir well.

6. Serve over steamed rice.

Yield: 8 servings, 8 cups
One Serving = 1 cup

Calories: 304	Fiber: 5 g
Protein: 24 g	Cholesterol: 76 mg
Fat: 17 g	Sodium: 385 mg
Carbohydrate: 17 mg	Potassium: 642 mg

Exchange: 3 medium-fat meat
             3 vegetable

APPLE PIE SWEETENED WITH RAISINS AND DATES _____

A delicious ending to a meal. Try it warm with a dollop of ricotta cheese flavored with nutmeg.

Filling
 ½ **cup raisins**
 ½ **cup pitted and chopped dates**
 ¾ **cup water**
 4 cups peeled, cored, and thinly sliced apples (5 to 6 apples)
 1 teaspoon freshly squeezed lemon juice
 1 teaspoon vanilla
 1 teaspoon cinnamon
 ½ **teaspoon nutmeg**
 ¼ **cup all-purpose flour**

Pastry Crust
 2 cups all-purpose flour
 ⅔ **cup chilled margarine**
 4 tablespoons or less unsweetened apple juice

1. Combine raisins, dates, and water in a small saucepan. Cover and bring to a boil. Turn to low and simmer 10 minutes. Remove from the heat and cool. Purée in a food processor or blender until smooth.
2. Toss together sliced apples and remaining filling ingredients. Add raisin-date mixture and mix well. Refrigerate.
3. To prepare pastry, combine flour and margarine until evenly blended. Gradually add apple juice until the dough is soft. Roll two thirds of the crust out on a lightly floured surface to ⅛-inch thickness. Fit into a 9-inch pie pan, trimming off the excess pastry. Combine with remaining pastry, rolling out in the same way, and cut into ½-inch-wide strips.
4. Spoon filling into pie shell and top with pastry strips to make a lattice design. Place strips close together so pie filling will not dry out during baking. Flute the edges. Bake in a preheated 450°F oven for 10 minutes; reduce heat to 350°F and continue baking 40 minutes more or until apples are tender. Cool on a wire rack.

Yield: 10 servings
One Serving = ¹⁄₁₀ of 9-inch pie

Calories: 296
Protein: 3 g
Fat: 13 g
Carbohydrate: 44 g

Fiber: 3.8 g
Cholesterol: 0
Sodium: 164 mg
Potassium: 240 mg

Exchange: 2 starch/bread
1 fruit
2 fat

HEARTY WINTER SUPPER

Squash and Mushroom Soup
Snow Peas with Lemon
Roast Veal
California Wild Rice
Blueberry Cobbler

Recommended wine:

- a medium, full-bodied red wine, such as a French Bordeaux or Burgundy, or a California Merlot or aged Cabernet Sauvignon.

SQUASH AND MUSHROOM SOUP

Good with a topping of nonfat yogurt or sliced, toasted almonds.

2 medium acorn or butternut squash	½ teaspoon cumin
2½ cups water	½ teaspoon cinnamon
1 cup orange juice	¾ teaspoon ginger
2 tablespoons margarine	½ to ¾ teaspoon salt
½ cup chopped onion	Dash of cayenne pepper
1 medium clove garlic, crushed	½ cup sliced mushrooms
½ teaspoon coriander or 1 tablespoon chopped fresh cilantro	

1. Split the squash lengthwise and bake face down in a preheated 375°F oven for 30 minutes or until soft. (You can also cook the squash in a microwave oven for 10 to 12 minutes on high.) Cool the squash and scoop out the insides. You should have approximately 3 cups of cooked squash.

2. Put the cooked squash and water in a blender or food processor and purée until smooth. Transfer to a soup pot and add the orange juice.

3. Heat the margarine in a skillet and add the onion, garlic, and seasonings. Sauté until the onion is soft, adding water if necessary to prevent sticking. Add mushrooms, cover, and cook for 10 minutes.

4. Add the sautéed mixture to the squash. Heat, stirring gently.

5. Taste to correct seasonings. Let simmer for 30 minutes or more to blend the flavors.

Yield: 6 servings, 6 cups
One Serving = 1 cup

Calories: 130	Fiber: 5 g*
Protein: 2 g	Cholesterol: 0
Fat: 6 g	Sodium: 376 mg
Carbohydrate: 20 g	Potassium: 399 mg

Exchange: 1 starch/bread
              1 fat

*Good source of dietary fiber

SNOW PEAS WITH LEMON ———————————— QUICK

2 cups or ¾ pound snow peas
1 teaspoon margarine
Zest of 1 large lemon
1 lemon slice for garnish

1. Steam snow peas until tender.

2. Toss peas with margarine and lemon rind.

3. Garnish with lemon slice and serve.

Yield: 4 servings, 2 cups
One Serving = ½ cup

Calories: 39	Fiber: 1.8 g
Protein: 2 g	Cholesterol: 0
Fat: 1 g	Sodium: 16 mg
Carbohydrate: 6 g	Potassium: 145 mg

Exchange: 1 vegetable

ROAST VEAL

1 tablespoon finely chopped rosemary leaves or 1 teaspoon dried
1 tablespoon finely chopped fresh sage or 1 teaspoon dried
3 cloves garlic, finely chopped
1 teaspoon coarse salt
Freshly ground black pepper to taste
1 3-pound round veal roast
1 tablespoon vegetable oil
3 tablespoons olive oil
1 to 1½ cups dry white wine

1. Preheat oven to 325°F.
2. Mix first 5 ingredients in a bowl. Cut 30 ½-inch-deep pockets in veal, spacing evenly. Press about ¼ teaspoon seasoning mixture into each. (You can prepare recipe up to this point, 1 day ahead. Cover and refrigerate.)
3. Place veal in a roasting pan slightly larger than the meat. Mix oils; pour over veal. Roast 1 hour, turning and basting veal with its juices every 20 minutes.
4. Add ½ cup wine to the roasting pan and cook until a meat thermometer inserted in the center registers 150°F, about 20 to 40 minutes more. As the veal cooks, you may have to add another ½ cup wine if liquid evaporates. Transfer veal to a platter. Tent with foil to keep warm and let stand 20 minutes.
5. Degrease the pan juices by skimming fat from the surface. Transfer juices to a small saucepan and set over high heat. Add ½ cup wine and bring to a boil. Boil until juices are thickened slightly, about 5 minutes. Slice veal and arrange on a platter. Pour sauce over veal and serve.

Yield: 10 servings
One Serving = 4 ounces

Calories: 217
Protein: 32 g
Fat: 9 g
Carbohydrate: <1 g

Fiber: 0
Cholesterol: 136 mg
Sodium: 217 mg
Potassium: 315 mg

Exchange: 4 lean meat

CALIFORNIA WILD RICE

½ pound (1⅜ cups) uncooked
  wild rice
5½ cups Chicken Stock (p. 290)
½ cup pecan halves
½ cup golden raisins
4 green onions, thinly sliced

2 tablespoons grated orange peel
2 tablespoons olive oil
⅓ cup orange juice
1 tablespoon chopped fresh mint
  or ½ teaspoon dried
Freshly ground black pepper to
  taste

1. Rinse rice under cold water. Simmer rice and chicken stock, covered, for 45 minutes. Drain.
2. Add pecans, raisins, and onions. Blend orange peel, olive oil, orange juice, mint, and pepper. Toss with rice.
3. Let stand 2 hours. Serve at room temperature.

Yield: 10 servings, 5 cups
One Serving = ½ cup

Calories: 204
Protein: 7 g
Fat: 7 g
Carbohydrate: 30 g

Fiber: 3.2 g
Cholesterol: 0
Sodium: 111 mg
Potassium: 322 mg

Exchange: 1 starch/bread
         1 fruit
         1½ fat

BLUEBERRY COBBLER ———————————————— QUICK

Warm and tender berries topped with sweetened biscuits. Serve straight from the oven.

  2 tablespoons sugar
  1½ tablespoons cornstarch
  1 cup unsweetened or freshly squeezed orange juice
  1½ cups frozen unsweetened blueberries, thawed
  1 teaspoon grated orange peel

Biscuits
  1 cup all-purpose flour
  1 teaspoon baking powder
  ¼ teaspoon baking soda
  ½ cup low-fat buttermilk
  1 tablespoon vegetable oil
  2 teaspoons sugar

1. Preheat oven to 375°F.
2. In a medium saucepan, combine 2 tablespoons sugar and corn-starch. Gradually stir in orange juice.
3. Cook over medium heat until mixture comes to a boil and is slightly thickened, stirring constantly.
4. Stir in blueberries and cook until fruit is hot. Stir in orange peel; set aside.
5. In a medium bowl, combine flour, baking powder, and baking soda.
6. Stir in buttermilk and oil just until dry ingredients are moistened.
7. Pour hot fruit mixture into an ungreased 1½-quart casserole. Drop dough by tablespoons over fruit mixture, keeping dough far enough apart to form 8 separate biscuits.
8. Sprinkle dough with 2 teaspoons sugar.
9. Bake for 20 to 25 minutes or until biscuits are light golden brown.

Yield: 8 servings, 2 cups berries, 8 biscuits
One Serving = ¼ cup berries with 1 biscuit

Calories: 121	Fiber: 1 g
Protein: 2 g	Cholesterol: 0.6 mg
Fat: 2 g	Sodium: 85 mg
Carbohydrate: 24 g	Potassium: 115 mg

Exchange: ½ starch/bread
            1 fruit

DINNER PARTY FOR SIX

Endive and Watercress Salad
Miniature Artichoke Hearts in Vinaigrette
Shrimp and Feta à la Grecque
Fresh sourdough bread with Creamy Cheese Spread
Melon with Slivered Almonds and Ginger

Recommended wine:

- a rich, full-bodied Chardonnay of high acidity to counteract feta cheese, such as a Chablis from France or an American Chardonnay
- a light, spicy red wine with good fruit such as a Pinot Noir from California or Oregon

ENDIVE AND WATERCRESS SALAD ———————— QUICK

4 medium Belgian endive or 2 small heads butterhead lettuce, sliced into rings ½ inch thick
1 cup watercress, well washed, thick stems removed
6 tablespoons Traditional Vinaigrette Dressing (p. 153)
2 tablespoons chopped walnuts

1. Mix together endive and watercress. Chill.
2. Just before serving, toss with dressing and top with walnuts.

Yield: 6 servings
One Serving = 1 cup salad and 1 tablespoon vinaigrette

Calories: 134
Protein: 3 g
Fat: 12 g
Carbohydrate: 6 g

Fiber: 5 g
Cholesterol: 0
Sodium: 91 mg
Potassium: 575 mg

Exchange: 1 vegetable
        2 fat

MINIATURE ARTICHOKE HEARTS IN VINAIGRETTE _____

Our light marinade for artichoke hearts is easy to make and will keep for weeks stored in a tightly covered jar.

1½ pounds artichokes (2-inch diameter)	1 teaspoon salt
3 cups water	1 teaspoon whole black peppercorns
⅓ cup red wine vinegar	4 to 5 cloves garlic, peeled and halved
⅓ cup olive oil	

1. Trim the artichokes by cutting off the tips and the end of the stems. Using scissors or a paring knife, remove any tough outer leaves. Depending on their size, you may want to halve or quarter the artichokes.

2. Put the artichokes in a saucepan with the other ingredients. Bring to a boil; then lower heat to medium. Continue to simmer for 40 minutes, or until the liquid is reduced to about 1 cup and the artichokes are tender.

3. Remove from heat and cool to room temperature. Serve immediately or store in the refrigerator in a jar with a tight-fitting lid.

Variation
Substitute 18 ounces frozen artichoke hearts for the fresh. Reduce the cooking time by about half.

Yield: 6 servings, 3 cups
One Serving = ½ cup

Calories: 40	Fiber: 1 g
Protein: 1 g	Cholesterol: 0
Fat: 2 g	Sodium: 55 mg
Carbohydrate: 6 g	Potassium: 221 mg

Exchange: 1 vegetable
      ½ fat

SHRIMP AND FETA À LA GRECQUE _____

> 4 tablespoons olive oil
> 1¼ pounds medium shrimp (about 36), shelled and deveined
> ¼ teaspoon red pepper flakes
> 1 small clove garlic, finely chopped
> ½ cup dry white wine
> 2 cups peeled and cubed tomatoes
> ⅓ cup chopped fresh basil or 2 tablespoons dried
> 2 teaspoons chopped fresh oregano or 1 teaspoon dried
> ⅛ teaspoon salt (optional)
> Freshly ground black pepper to taste
> 6 ounces feta cheese, crumbled
> 12 ounces fettuccine
> 1 tablespoon olive oil

1. Preheat oven to 400°F.

2. Heat 2 tablespoons of the olive oil in a skillet. Sauté shrimp just until they turn pink. Stir in the red pepper flakes. Transfer shrimp and pan juices to a baking dish.

3. Add remaining oil to the skillet. Briefly sauté the garlic. Add the wine and cook for 2 minutes over high heat.

4. Stir in tomatoes, basil, oregano, salt (if desired), and pepper. Simmer, uncovered, for 10 minutes.

5. Sprinkle the feta cheese over the shrimp. Spoon the tomato sauce over all. Cover dish and bake for 10 minutes.

6. Cook fettuccine in a large pot of boiling water until tender but still firm (about 8 minutes). Drain, toss with olive oil, and transfer to a serving bowl. Add shrimp-tomato mixture and gently mix with fettuccine. Serve immediately.

Yield: 6 servings, 8 cups
One Serving = 1½ cups

Calories: 387
Protein: 18 g
Fat: 19 g
Carbohydrate: 37 g

Fiber: 1 g
Cholesterol: 81 mg
Sodium: 349 mg (without salt)
Potassium: 247 mg

Exchange: 2 starch/bread
2 lean meat
1 vegetable
2 fat

CREAMY CHEESE SPREAD

This is a wonderful substitute for using butter on bread at meals.

1 cup low-fat cottage cheese
3 tablespoons margarine
1 tablespoon nonfat milk

Mix all ingredients in a blender or food processor until smooth.

Yield: 16 servings, 1 cup
One Serving = 1 tablespoon

Calories: 32	Fiber: 0
Protein: 2 g	Cholesterol: 1 mg
Fat: 2 g	Sodium: 86 mg
Carbohydrate: 1 g	Potassium: 16 mg

Exchange: ½ fat

MELON WITH SLIVERED ALMONDS AND GINGER — QUICK

2 cups peeled, seeded, and cubed cantaloupe
4 tablespoons toasted, slivered almonds
1 cup seedless green grapes
½ teaspoon finely minced ginger root
1 tablespoon freshly squeezed lime juice

Mix all ingredients together. Chill and serve.

Yield: 6 servings, 3 cups
One Serving = ½ cup

Calories: 72	Fiber: 1.1 g
Protein: 2 g	Cholesterol: 0
Fat: 3 g	Sodium: 7 mg
Carbohydrate: 11 g	Potassium: 261 mg

Exchange: 1 fruit
          ½ fat

SUMMER SEAFOOD BOUNTY

Spinach Dill Phyllo Triangles
San Diego Cioppino
Black rye bread with Creamy Cheese Spread (p. 322)
Watermelon Ice

Recommended wine:

- a full-bodied white wine, such as a Chardonnay from California
- a lighter spicy red wine, such as a California Pinot Noir or French Burgundy

SPINACH DILL PHYLLO TRIANGLES

Filling

2 packages (10 ounces each) frozen chopped spinach
1 cup finely chopped onion
2 tablespoons olive oil
¼ teaspoon nutmeg
½ teaspoon freshly ground black pepper
1 cup finely chopped fresh dill weed
⅔ cup part-skim ricotta cheese
½ cup crumbled feta cheese

Pastry

1 pound phyllo dough (available at Greek and Middle Eastern food stores and some delis)
½ cup melted margarine

1. To prepare filling, defrost the frozen spinach, drain, and squeeze out as much remaining moisture as possible.
2. Sauté the onion in olive oil until golden, about 20 minutes. Add the spinach and cook over low heat, stirring constantly, for 10 to 15 minutes, or until mixture is dry. Season with nutmeg and pepper and let cool.
3. Transfer spinach mixture to a bowl and stir in dill, ricotta, and feta, mixing well.

4. To make pastry, unwrap the phyllo dough, unroll it, and cover it immediately with a towel to keep it from drying out. Let it stand for 15 minutes before working with it.

5. Uncover the dough and cut the phyllo sheets into thirds, lengthwise, with a sharp knife.

6. Remove 1 strip and cover the rest of the pastry. Brush strip with margarine, fold in half, and brush again with a small amount of additional margarine.

7. Place a heaping teaspoon of filling in a corner of the strip and fold the strip in a triangular shape, as if you were folding a flag. Tuck any excess under the triangle and brush with margarine again. Repeat with remaining filling and dough.

8. Place triangles on a lightly oiled baking sheet. (You can refrigerate triangles for up to 24 hours before baking.)

9. Bake in a preheated 350°F oven for about 25 minutes or until triangles are well browned and filling is hot. Serve immediately.

Yield: 30 servings, approximately 30 triangles, 4 cups filling
One Serving = 1 triangle

Calories: 64	Fiber: 0.8 g
Protein: 2 g	Cholesterol: 13 mg
Fat: 4 g	Sodium: 76 mg
Carbohydrate: 5 g	Potassium: 78 mg

Exchange: 1 vegetable
          1 fat

SAN DIEGO CIOPPINO

2 freshly cooked whole crabs, approximately 2 pounds each, or 4 1-pound cocktail-size crab claws
12 clams, well scrubbed
12 mussels, well scrubbed
3 cups dry white wine
¼ cup olive oil
1 medium onion, finely chopped
4 cloves garlic, minced
1 medium green pepper, coarsely chopped
2 pounds tomatoes, peeled, seeded, and chopped
3 ounces tomato paste
1 teaspoon freshly ground black pepper
½ teaspoon oregano
1 tablespoon finely chopped fresh basil or ½ teaspoon dried
2 pounds fresh white fish such as sea bass, rock cod, red snapper, or halibut, cut into large pieces
¾ pound scallops
¾ pound shrimp, shelled and deveined
Chopped fresh parsley and sun-dried tomatoes for garnish

1. If using whole crab, remove legs and claws from the body and break the body in half. Set aside.

2. Place the clams and mussels in a pan, add 1 cup of the wine, and steam, covered, over medium heat for 5 to 6 minutes or until clams and mussels open. Remove shellfish, discarding any that do not open. Strain the stock through cheesecloth and save.

3. In an 8-quart casserole or kettle, heat the oil. Add the onion, garlic, and green pepper, and sauté over medium heat, stirring occasionally, until the vegetables start to soften, about 5 minutes.

4. Add tomatoes, tomato paste, the remaining 2 cups of wine, pepper, herbs, and clam stock. Partially cover and simmer for 20 minutes. Add the fish, scallops, shrimp, and crabs or crab claws. Simmer for approximately 5 minutes or until all the seafood is cooked. Do not stir. Add the clams and mussels and heat for 1 minute.

5. Sprinkle with parsley and sun-dried tomatoes and serve immediately from the cooking pot.

Yield: 8 servings, about 12 cups
One Serving = 1½ cups

Calories: 349
Protein: 52 g
Fat: 10 g
Carbohydrate: 12 g

Fiber: 2.5 g
Cholesterol: 194 mg
Sodium: 497 mg*
Potassium: 1199 mg

Exchange: 5½ lean meat
           2 vegetable

*High in sodium

WATERMELON ICE

1 teaspoon unflavored gelatin
4 cups watermelon cubes
2 tablespoons freshly squeezed lime juice
2 tablespoons honey
Lime twists for garnish

1. In a small nonstick saucepan, soften gelatin in 2 tablespoons water over medium heat. Stir until gelatin is dissolved.
2. In a blender container, combine 1 cup of the melon cubes, lime juice, honey, and gelatin mixture. Cover and blend at high speed for 30 seconds or until smooth.
3. Add remaining melon in batches; cover and blend at high speed for 30 to 45 seconds or until smooth.
4. Pour into an 8 × 8 × 2-inch pan and freeze until almost firm.
5. Remove from freezer and transfer mixture to a large chilled bowl. Beat at high speed with an electric mixer or food processor until smooth. Return to the pan and freeze for several hours or until firm.
6. To serve, let stand for 15 to 20 minutes at room temperature. Scrape surface and spoon into serving dishes. If desired, garnish with lime twists.

Yield: 6 servings, 6 cups
One Serving = 1 cup

Calories: 58
Protein: 1 g
Fat: <1 g
Carbohydrate: 14 g

Fiber: 0.5 g
Cholesterol: 0
Sodium: 4 mg
Potassium: 133 mg

Exchange: 1 fruit

HOLIDAY FEAST

Sparkling Fall Harvest Punch
Spinach-Stuffed Mushrooms
Herb-Roasted Turkey with Traditional Onion-Herb
    Stuffing
Asparagus with Creamy Orange Sauce
Apple Oatmeal Muffins
Pumpkin Mousse Pie

Recommended wine:

- a spicy California Gewürztraminer or German Riesling
- a Pinot Noir from Oregon or California

SPARKLING FALL HARVEST PUNCH —————— EASY

2 cups cranberry juice
2 cups apple juice
1½ cups orange juice

2 cups club soda
Orange slices and cranberries for
    garnish

1. Combine juices in a large bowl or pitcher.
2. Just before serving, add club soda and stir. Garnish with sliced oranges and fresh whole cranberries.

Yield: 10 servings, 7½ cups
One Serving = ¾ cup

Calories: 71
Protein: <1 g
Fat: trace
Carbohydrate: 17 g

Fiber: 0.1 g
Cholesterol: 0
Sodium: 13 mg
Potassium: 146 mg

Exchange: 1 fruit

SPINACH-STUFFED MUSHROOMS _____

6 mushrooms, 2 inches in
   diameter
Nonstick vegetable spray
½ pound spinach leaves, cleaned,
   stems removed
1 clove garlic, minced

2 egg whites
1 tablespoon margarine
1 tablespoon all-purpose flour
2 tablespoons freshly grated
   Parmesan cheese

1. Clean mushrooms and remove stems; reserve for other uses.
2. Coat a baking dish with nonstick spray and arrange mushrooms cut side up. Set aside.
3. Cook spinach in frying pan over medium heat until wilted (about 3 minutes).
4. Mix garlic and egg whites in a blender or food processor until frothy. Add spinach and blend until puréed.
5. Melt margarine in skillet, add flour, and cook, stirring, until bubbly.
6. Remove from heat and stir in spinach mixture.
7. Spoon equal amounts of spinach mixture into each mushroom cap. Sprinkle evenly with Parmesan cheese.
8. Bake uncovered in a preheated 400°F oven for 10 to 15 minutes or until cheese is golden and filling is puffy.
9. Serve immediately.

Yield: 3 servings, 6 mushrooms
One Serving = 2 mushrooms

Calories: 100
Protein: 7 g
Fat: 5 g
Carbohydrate: 8 g

Fiber: 4.1 g
Cholesterol: 3 mg
Sodium: 159 mg
Potassium: 657 mg

Exchange: 2 vegetable
        1 fat

HERB-ROASTED TURKEY ———————————

Very quick and easy, especially if you use the microwave!

> 3½ to 4 pounds boneless turkey breast
> 2 large garlic cloves, thinly sliced
> ½ teaspoon salt
> 1 tablespoon chopped fresh rosemary or 1 teaspoon dried
> 2 teaspoons chopped fresh thyme or ½ teaspoon dried
> Paprika
> 4 green onions, trimmed of ends and tops

1. Rinse turkey and pat dry. Loosen lining under skin with a knife. Pull skin back, leaving it attached along one edge.
2. Make cuts in surface of turkey and insert garlic slices. Combine salt and herbs. Sprinkle turkey with half the mixture. Replace skin and secure with toothpicks.
3. Sprinkle turkey with remaining herb mixture and paprika.
4. Place turkey in a roasting pan. Fold green onions in half lengthwise and place inside the cavity of the turkey breast.
5. Bake in a preheated 325°F oven for 2 to 2½ hours to an internal temperature of 170°F or until meat is no longer pink. Let stand 10 minutes before slicing.

Microwave
1. Prepare turkey as described in steps 1 through 3. Place in a glass baking dish, skin side down.
2. Cover with plastic wrap, turning back one corner to vent. Cook in microwave on high for 11 minutes. Turn skin side up and place onions underneath breast. Cook for an additional 20 to 30 minutes. Total cooking time should be approximately 7 to 10 minutes per pound of turkey.

Yield: 10 to 12 servings
One Serving = 3 ounces

Calories: 154	Fiber: 0.2 g
Protein: 28 g	Cholesterol: 71 mg
Fat: 4 g	Sodium: 154 mg
Carbohydrate: <1 g	Potassium: 269 mg

Exchange: 3 lean meat

TRADITIONAL ONION-HERB STUFFING _____

3 cups fresh whole wheat bread
  crumbs
1½ cups coarsely chopped
  mushrooms
1 cup finely chopped celery
2 cups finely chopped onions

1 teaspoon thyme
1 teaspoon sage
¼ teaspoon finely ground black
  pepper
¼ to ½ cup water or Chicken
  Stock (p. 290)

1. In a large bowl, combine all ingredients.
2. Bake in a covered casserole dish in a preheated 325°F oven for approximately 40 minutes.

Yield: 6 servings, 6 cups
One Serving = 1 cup

Calories: 65
Protein: 3 g
Fat: <1 g
Carbohydrate: 13 g

Fiber: 1.5 g
Cholesterol: 0
Sodium: 102 mg
Potassium: 175 mg

Exchange: 1 starch/bread

ASPARAGUS WITH CREAMY ORANGE SAUCE _____ QUICK

1½ pounds asparagus
½ cup reduced-calorie
  mayonnaise
3 tablespoons nonfat milk

1 teaspoon grated orange peel
1 tablespoon freshly squeezed
  orange juice
Dash of Tabasco sauce

1. Break off tough ends of the asparagus and discard. Steam the asparagus, covered, for approximately 6 minutes or until barely tender. Drain and place on a serving platter. Keep warm.
2. In a small saucepan, combine mayonnaise, milk, orange peel, juice, and Tabasco. Stir until well blended.
3. Cook sauce over very low heat for about 3 minutes or until thoroughly heated, stirring constantly so sauce does not burn. Serve immediately, over asparagus or on the side.

Yield: 6 servings, 3 cups asparagus, ¾ cup sauce
One Serving = ½ cup asparagus, 2 tablespoons sauce

Calories: 98
Protein: 3 g
Fat: 7 g
Carbohydrate: 7 g

Fiber: 1.4 g
Cholesterol: 3 mg
Sodium: 169 mg
Potassium: 369 mg

Exchange: 1 vegetable
            1½ fat

APPLE OATMEAL MUFFINS

A good source of soluble fiber.

Nonstick vegetable spray
¾ cup old-fashioned or quick oats
¼ cup oat bran
½ cup all-purpose flour
3 tablespoons brown sugar
2 teaspoons baking powder
⅛ teaspoon salt

1 teaspoon cinnamon
½ cup unsweetened apple juice
¼ cup low-fat milk
1 egg
2 tablespoons vegetable oil
1 medium apple, grated
2 tablespoons raisins

1. Preheat oven to 400°F.
2. Grease a 12-cup muffin tin with nonstick spray.
3. Combine oats, oat bran, flour, brown sugar, baking powder, salt, and cinnamon; set aside.
4. In a large mixing bowl, combine apple juice, milk, egg, and oil.
5. Add dry ingredients to liquids. Stir in apple and raisins until just moistened. Do not overmix.
6. Fill muffin tin and bake for about 20 minutes or until muffins are golden brown and a cake tester comes out clean.

Yield: 12 muffins
One Serving = 1 muffin

Calories: 105
Protein: 2 g
Fat: 3 g
Carbohydrate: 17 g

Fiber: 1.3 g
Cholesterol: 23 mg
Sodium: 81 mg
Potassium: 106 mg

Exchange: 1 starch/bread
            ½ fat

PUMPKIN MOUSSE PIE ——————————————— EASY

10 vanilla wafers, crushed
1 tablespoon margarine, melted
1 package unflavored gelatin
1½ cups evaporated skim milk
¾ cup part-skim ricotta cheese
1 cup canned pumpkin
10 to 12 packages Equal
1 teaspoon vanilla
½ tablespoon pumpkin pie spice
1 envelope reduced-calorie whipped topping mix

Crust

In a blender or food processor, crush vanilla wafers. Mix with melted margarine and press into an ungreased pie plate and freeze for 1 hour.

Filling

1. Sprinkle gelatin over ½ cup evaporated milk. Let stand 10 minutes; gently heat until gelatin dissolves.
2. In a blender or food processor, blend milk-gelatin mixture with ricotta cheese, pumpkin, Equal, vanilla, pumpkin pie spice, and remaining milk. Pour into pie crust and chill.

Topping

Prepare whipped topping according to package directions and spoon a dollop onto each slice of pie.

Yield: 8 servings
One Serving = ⅛ pie

Calories: 127
Protein: 8 g
Fat: 4 g
Carbohydrate: 15 g

Fiber: trace
Cholesterol: 12 mg
Sodium: 118 mg
Potassium: 280 mg

Exchange: 1 starch/bread
1 lean meat

COLD BUFFET LUNCHEON

Salade Niçoise
Basil Rolls
Black-and-White Meringues with Strawberries in
    Balsamic Vinegar

Recommended wine:

- a champagne or sparkling wine from California
- a zippy white wine such as an American Sauvignon Blanc or French Provençale rosé

SALADE NIÇOISE

This recipe is adapted from one of the all-time favorites served at Café Champagne, at the Culbertson Winery in Temecula, California.

Dressing

¼ cup corn oil
¼ cup olive oil
¼ cup champagne or white wine
    vinegar
2 cloves garlic, crushed

1 to 2 tablespoons fresh basil or ½
    teaspoon dried
¼ teaspoon salt
⅛ teaspoon freshly ground black
    pepper

Salad

About 6 cups assorted lettuce, washed and broken into bite-size pieces
6 new red potatoes, cooked and sliced
¾ pound baby green beans, blanched
18 ounces fresh grilled tuna*
2 tomatoes cut into 12 wedges

1. Toss the salad greens with the dressing and cover about a third of the plate with them.
2. Toss the potatoes and green beans separately in the dressing and arrange on the plate.
3. Grill the tuna and cut in thin slices. Serve immediately and garnish with tomato wedges.

*Substitute an equal amount of low-sodium, water-packed, white albacore tuna if fresh tuna is not available.

Yield: 6 servings
One Serving = 1½ cups salad with 3 ounces tuna

Calories: 408
Protein: 27 g
Fat: 19 g
Carbohydrate: 23 g

Fiber: 2.2 g
Cholesterol: 51 mg
Sodium: 130 mg
Potassium: 829 mg

Exchange: 3 lean meat
2 fat
1 starch/bread
2 vegetable

BASIL ROLLS

Cottage cheese makes these rolls moist and provides additional calcium and protein. They make a wonderful accompaniment to soup or salad.

1 package active dry yeast
1 teaspoon honey
½ to ¾ cup warm water (110°F)
1 cup low-fat cottage cheese
½ cup chopped fresh basil or 2 tablespoons dried
1 egg
2 teaspoons baking powder
¼ teaspoon baking soda
1 teaspoon salt
3½ to 4 cups unbleached all-purpose or whole wheat flour
2 tablespoons margarine
1 tablespoon freshly grated Parmesan cheese

1. In a small bowl, dissolve yeast and honey in water. Let stand until bubbly. Combine cottage cheese, basil, and egg until smooth.
2. In a large bowl, stir together baking powder, baking soda, salt, and 3¼ cups flour.
3. Work margarine into flour mixture with fingers until evenly distributed.
4. Stir in cottage cheese mixture and yeast.
5. Turn dough onto a floured board and knead until smooth (approximately 10 minutes), adding flour as needed to prevent sticking.

6. Place dough in lightly oiled bowl, cover, and let rise until doubled in size, about 30 minutes.

7. Punch down dough. Divide into 18 equal pieces. Roll into ball shape and arrange in 2 nonstick 8-inch round baking pans. Cover and let rise about 10 minutes.

8. Brush tops of rolls lightly with water and sprinkle with Parmesan cheese.

9. Bake in 350°F oven for 25 minutes or until crust is golden brown. Cool on racks.

Yield: 18 rolls
One Serving = 1 roll

Calories: 121	Fiber: 2.6 g
Protein: 6 g	Cholesterol: 16 mg
Fat: 2 g	Sodium: 227 mg
Carbohydrate: 20 g	Potassium: 139 mg

Exchange: 1½ starch/bread

BLACK-AND-WHITE MERINGUES _____ QUICK

This recipe is slightly higher in simple sugar content than what we would generally recommend, but it makes a very special dessert. Combine it with our low-fat Whipped Topping (p. 297) or serve with berries or custard.

3 egg whites at room temperature	1 teaspoon vanilla
⅛ teaspoon cream of tartar	2 tablespoons unsweetened cocoa
3 teaspoons fructose	powder

1. Whip the egg whites and cream of tartar with an electric beater until stiff but not dry. Gradually add half of the fructose.
2. Combine vanilla with 2 teaspoons water. Add the liquid to the egg whites, a few drops at a time, alternately with the remaining fructose, whipping constantly.
3. Remove a third of the batter and set aside. Fold cocoa into the remaining batter.
4. Drop a sixth of the cocoa batter from a spoon onto a nonstick baking sheet (or one that you have covered with waxed paper). Repeat until there are 6 rounds, and top each with a dollop of white meringue batter. Make a large hollow in the center of each meringue, using the back of a spoon.
5. Bake meringues in a preheated 250°F oven for approximately 30 minutes or until firm to the touch and lightly browned. Cool on a wire rack.
6. Fill meringues with berries, topping, or custard shortly before serving.

Yield: 6 servings, 6 3-inch meringues
One Serving = 1 meringue

Calories: 23	Fiber: 0
Protein: 2 g	Cholesterol: 0
Fat: <1 g	Sodium: 25 mg
Carbohydrate: 3 g	Potassium: 52 mg

Exchange: Free

STRAWBERRIES IN BALSAMIC VINEGAR ——————— EASY

Balsamic vinegar, from Italy, is aged for at least ten years in wooden barrels. It is a deep reddish-brown, full-bodied, and slightly sweet in flavor. You can find it in specialty or gourmet shops, as well as in some grocery stores. It imparts a special flavor to fresh strawberries.

2 pints (4 cups) fresh strawberries
2 to 3 packages Equal
1 tablespoon balsamic vinegar

1. Wash and hull the strawberries.
2. Halve or slice the berries, depending on the size and your personal preference. Place them in a shallow pan and sprinkle with Equal.
3. Cover container tightly with plastic wrap and let sit for several hours. Stir the strawberries occasionally. If they sit for more than 3 hours, refrigerate, but allow them to return to room temperature before serving.
4. Sprinkle berries with vinegar ½ hour or less before serving.

Yield: 6 servings, 4 cups
One Serving = ¾ cup

Calories: 36
Protein: 1 g
Fat: <1 g
Carbohydrate: 8 g

Fiber: 2.1 g
Cholesterol: 0
Sodium: 1 mg
Potassium: 167 mg

Exchange: ½ fruit

APPENDIX

Exchange Lists for Meal Planning

STARCH/BREAD LIST

Each item in this list contains approximately 15 grams of carbohydrate, 3 grams of protein, a trace of fat, and 80 calories. Whole grain products average about 2 grams of fiber per serving. Some foods are higher in fiber. Those foods that contain 3 or more grams of fiber per serving are identified with an asterisk (*).

You can choose your starch exchanges from any of the items on this list. If you want to eat a starch food that is not on the list, the general rule is that:

- ½ cup of cereal, grain, or pasta is one serving
- 1 ounce of a bread product is one serving

Your dietitian can help you be more exact.

Cereals, Grains, and Pasta

*Bran cereals, concentrated	⅓ c
*Bran cereals, flaked (such as Bran Buds, All Bran)	½ c
Bulgur (cooked)	½ c

*Indicates 3 g or more of fiber

Cooked cereals	½ c
Cornmeal	2½ T
Grapenuts	3 T
Grits (cooked)	½ c
Other ready-to-eat unsweetened cereals	¾ c
Pasta (cooked)	½ c
Puffed cereal	1½ c
Rice, white or brown (cooked)	⅓ c
Shredded wheat	½ c
*Wheat germ	3 T

Dried Beans, Peas, and Lentils

*Baked beans	¼ c
*Beans and peas (cooked), such as kidney, white, split, black-eyed	⅓ c
*Lentils (cooked)	⅓ c

Starchy Vegetables

*Corn	½ c
*Corn on cob, 6 in. long	1
*Lima beans	½ c
*Peas, green (canned or frozen)	½ c
*Plantain	½ c
Potato, baked	1 small (3 oz)
Potato, mashed	½ c
*Squash, winter (acorn, butternut)	¾ c
Yam, sweet potato	⅓ c

Bread

Bagel	½ (1 oz)
Bread sticks, crisp, 4 in. long × ½ in.	2 (⅔ oz)
Croutons, low-fat	1 c
English muffin	½
Frankfurter or hamburger bun	½ (1 oz)
Pita, 6 in. across	½
Plain roll, small	1 (1 oz)
Raisin	1 slice (1 oz)
Rye, pumpernickel	1 slice (1 oz)

*Indicates 3 g or more of fiber

Tortilla, 6 in. across	1
White (including French, Italian)	1 slice (1 oz)
Whole wheat	1 slice (1 oz)

Crackers, Snacks

Animal crackers	8
Graham crackers, 2½ in. square	3
Matzoth	¾ oz
Melba toast	5 slices
Oyster crackers	24
Popcorn (popped, no fat added)	3 c
Pretzels	¾ oz
RyKrisp, 2 in. × 3½ in.	4
Saltines	6
Whole wheat crackers, no fat added (crisp breads, such as Finn, Kavli, Wasa)	2–4 slices (¾ oz)

Starch Foods Prepared with Fat

(Count as 1 starch/bread serving, plus 1 fat serving.)

Biscuit, 2½ in. across	1
Chow mein noodles	½ c
Corn bread, 2 in. square	1 (2 oz)
Cracker, round butter	6
French-fried potatoes, 2 in. to 3½ in. long	10 (1½ oz)
Muffin, plain, small	1
Pancake, 4 in. across	2
Stuffing, bread (prepared)	¼ c
Taco shell, 6 in. across	2
Waffle, 4½ in. square	1
Whole wheat crackers, fat added (such as Triscuits)	4–6 (1 oz)

MEAT LIST

Each serving of meat and substitutes in this list contains about 7 grams of protein. The amount of fat and number of calories vary, depending on what kind of meat or substitute you choose. The list is divided into three parts based on the amount of fat and calories: lean meat, medium-fat meat, and high-fat meat. One ounce (one meat exchange) of each of these includes:

	Carbohydrate (grams)	Protein (grams)	Fat (grams)	Calories
Lean	0	7	3	55
Medium-Fat	0	7	5	75
High-Fat	0	7	8	100

We encourage you to use more lean and medium-fat meat, poultry, and fish in your meal plan. This will help decrease your fat intake, which may help decrease your risk for heart disease. The items from the high-fat group are high in saturated fat, cholesterol, and calories. You should limit your choices from the high-fat group to three times per week. Meat and substitutes do not contribute any fiber to your meal plan. Meats and meat substitutes that have 400 milligrams or more of sodium per exchange are indicated by a dagger (†).

TIPS

1. Bake, roast, broil, grill, or boil these foods rather than frying them with added fat.
2. Use a nonstick vegetable spray or a nonstick pan to brown or fry these foods.
3. Trim off visible fat before and after cooking.
4. Do not add flour, bread crumbs, coating mixes, or fat to these foods when preparing them.
5. Weigh meat after removing bones and fat, and after cooking. Three ounces of cooked meat is about equal to 4 ounces of raw meat. Some examples of meat portions are:
    2 ounces meat (2 meat exchanges) =
       1 small chicken leg or thigh
       ½ cup cottage cheese or tuna
    3 ounces meat (3 meat exchanges) =
       1 medium pork chop
       1 small hamburger
       ½ of a whole chicken breast
       1 unbreaded fish fillet
       cooked meat, about the size of a deck of cards
6. Restaurants usually serve Prime cuts of meat, which are high in fat and calories.

Lean Meat and Substitutes
(One exchange is equal to any one of the following items.)

Beef: USDA Good or Choice grades of lean beef, such   1 oz
as round, sirloin, and flank steak; tenderloin; and
†chipped beef

Pork: Lean pork, such as fresh ham; †canned, cured   1 oz
or boiled ham; †Canadian bacon, tenderloin

Veal: All cuts are lean except for veal cutlets (ground   1 oz
or cubed).

Poultry: Chicken, turkey, Cornish hen (without skin)   1 oz

Seafood: All fresh and frozen fish   1 oz

Crab, lobster, scallops, shrimp, clams (fresh or   2 oz
†canned in water)

Oysters   6 medium

†Tuna (canned in water)   ¼ c

Herring (uncreamed or smoked)   1 oz

Sardines (canned)   2 medium

Wild Game: Venison, rabbit, squirrel   1 oz

Pheasant, duck, goose (without skin)   1 oz

Cheese: Any cottage cheese   ¼ c

†Low-fat cheeses (with less than 55 calories per oz)   1 oz

Grated Parmesan   2 T

Other: 95% fat-free luncheon meat   1 oz

Egg whites   3

Egg substitutes with less than 55 calories per ¼ c   ¼ c

Medium-Fat Meat and Substitutes
(One exchange is equal to any one of the following items.)

Beef: Most beef products fall into this category: all   1 oz
ground beef, roast (rib, chuck, rump), steak (cubed,
Porterhouse, T-bone), and meat loaf.

Pork: Most pork products fall into this category.   1 oz
Examples are chops, loin roast, Boston butt,
cutlets.

†Indicates 400 mg or more of sodium

Lamb: Most lamb products fall into this category. Examples are chops, leg, and roast. — 1 oz

Veal: Cutlet (ground or cubed, unbreaded) — 1 oz

Poultry: Chicken (with skin), domestic duck or goose (well drained of fat), ground turkey — 1 oz

Seafood: †Tuna (canned in oil and drained) — ¼ c

†Salmon (canned) — ¼ c

Cheese: Skim or part-skim milk cheeses, such as:

Ricotta — ¼ c

Mozzarella — 1 oz

†Diet cheeses (with 56–80 calories per oz) — 1 oz

Other: †86% fat-free luncheon meat — 1 oz

Egg (high in cholesterol, limit to 3 per week) — 1

Egg substitutes with 56–80 calories per ¼ c — ¼ c

Tofu (2½ in. × 2¾ in. × 1 in.) — 4 oz

Liver, heart, kidney, sweetbreads (high in cholesterol) — 1 oz

High-Fat Meat and Substitutes

Remember, these items are high in saturated fat, cholesterol, and calories, and should be used only three times per week. (*One exchange is equal to any one of the following items.*)

Beef: Most USDA Prime cuts of beef, such as ribs, †corned beef — 1 oz

Pork: Spareribs, ground pork, †pork sausage (patty or link) — 1 oz

Lamb: Patties (ground lamb) — 1 oz

Seafood: Any fried fish product — 1 oz

Cheese: All regular †cheeses, such as American, Blue, Cheddar, Monterey Jack, Swiss — 1 oz

Other: †Luncheon meat, such as bologna, salami, pimiento loaf — 1 oz

†Sausage, such as Polish, Italian, or smoked — 1 oz

Knockwurst — 1 oz

†Indicates 400 mg or more of sodium

†Bratwurst	1 oz
†Frankfurter (turkey or chicken)	1 frank (10/lb)
Peanut butter (contains unsaturated fat)	1 T

Count as one high-fat meat plus one fat exchange:

| †Frankfurter (beef, pork, or combination) | 1 frank (10/lb) |

*VEGETABLE LIST

Each vegetable serving on this list contains about 5 grams of carbohydrate, 2 grams of protein, and 25 calories. Vegetables contain 2 to 3 grams of dietary fiber. Vegetables that contain 400 milligrams of sodium per serving are identified with a dagger (†).

Vegetables are a good source of vitamins and minerals. Fresh and frozen vegetables have more vitamins and less added salt than canned vegetables. Rinsing canned vegetables will remove much of the salt.

Unless otherwise noted, the serving size for vegetables (one vegetable exchange) is:

- ½ cup of cooked vegetables or vegetable juice
- 1 cup of raw vegetables

Artichoke (½ medium)
Asparagus
Beans (green, wax, Italian)
Bean sprouts
Beets
Broccoli
Brussels sprouts
Cabbage, cooked
Carrots
Cauliflower
Eggplant
Greens (collard, mustard, turnip)

*Indicates 3 g or more of fiber
†Indicates 400 mg or more of sodium

Kohlrabi

Leeks

Mushrooms, cooked

Okra

Onions

Pea pods

Peppers (green)

Rutabaga

†Sauerkraut

Spinach, cooked

Summer squash (crookneck)

Tomato (large)

†Tomato/vegetable juice

Turnips

Water chestnuts

Zucchini, cooked

Starchy vegetables such as corn, peas, and potatoes are found in the Starch/Bread List.

For free vegetables, see Free Foods List.

FRUIT LIST

Each item in this list contains about 15 grams of carbohydrate and 60 calories. Fresh, frozen, and dried fruits have about 2 grams of fiber per serving. An asterisk (*) indicates fruits that have 3 or more grams of fiber per serving. Fruit juices contain very little dietary fiber.

The carbohydrate and calorie content for a fruit serving are based on the usual serving of the most commonly eaten fruits. Use fresh fruits or fruits frozen or canned without sugar added. Whole fruit is more filling than fruit juice and may be a better choice if you

*Indicates 3 g or more of fiber
†Indicates 400 mg or more of sodium

are trying to lose weight. Unless otherwise noted, the serving size for one fruit serving is:

- ½ cup of fresh fruit or fruit juice
- ¼ cup of dried fruit

Fresh, Frozen, and Unsweetened Canned Fruit

Apple (raw, 2 in. across)	1 apple
Applesauce (unsweetened)	½ c
Apricots (medium, raw)	4 apricots
(canned)	½ c, or 4 halves
Banana (9 in. long)	½ banana
*Blackberries (raw)	¾ c
*Blueberries (raw)	¾ c
Cantaloupe (5 in. across)	⅓ melon
(cubes)	1 c
Cherries (large, raw)	12 cherries
(canned)	½ c
Figs (raw, 2 in. across)	2 figs
Fruit cocktail (canned)	½ c
Grapefruit (medium)	½ grapefruit
(segments)	¾ c
Grapes (small)	15 grapes
Honeydew melon (medium)	⅛ melon
(cubes)	1 c
Kiwi (large)	1 kiwi
Mandarin oranges	¾ c
Mango (small)	½ mango
*Nectarine (2½ in. across)	1 nectarine
Orange (2½ in. across)	1 orange
Papaya	1 c
Peach (2¾ in. across)	1 peach, or ¾ c
(canned)	½ c, or 2 halves
Pear	½ large, or 1 small
(canned)	½ c or 2 halves

*Indicates 3 g or more of fiber

Persimmon (medium, native)	2 persimmons
Pineapple (raw)	¾ c
(canned)	⅓ c
Plum (2 in. across)	2 plums
*Pomegranate	½ pomegranate
*Raspberries (raw)	1 c
*Strawberries (raw, whole)	1¼ c
Tangerine (2½ in. across)	2 tangerines
Watermelon (cubes)	1¼ c

Dried Fruit

*Apples	4 rings
*Apricots	7 halves
Dates	2½ medium
*Figs	1½
*Prunes	3 medium
Raisins	2 T

Fruit Juice

Apple juice/cider	½ c
Cranberry juice cocktail	⅓ c
Grapefruit juice	½ c
Grape juice	⅓ c
Orange juice	½ c
Pineapple juice	½ c
Prune juice	⅓ c

MILK LIST

Each serving of milk or milk products in this list contains about 12 grams of carbohydrate and 8 grams of protein. The amount of fat in milk is measured in percent of butterfat. The calories vary, depending on what kind of milk you choose. The list is divided into three parts based on the amount of fat and calories: skim/very low fat milk, low-fat milk, and whole milk. One serving (one milk exchange) of each of these includes:

*Indicates 3 g or more of fiber

	Carbohydrate (grams)	Protein (grams)	Fat (grams)	Calories
Skim/Very low fat	12	8	trace	90
Low-fat	12	8	5	120
Whole	12	8	8	150

Milk is the body's main source of calcium, the mineral needed for growth and repair of bones. Yogurt is also a good source of calcium. Yogurt and many dry or powdered milk products have different amounts of fat. If you have questions about a particular item, read the label to find out the fat and calorie content.

Milk is good to drink, but it can also be added to cereal, and to other foods. Many tasty dishes, such as sugar-free pudding, are made with milk (see the Combination Foods list). Add life to plain yogurt by adding one of your fruit servings to it.

Skim and Very Low Fat Milk

Skim milk	1 c
½% milk	1 c
1% milk	1 c
Low-fat buttermilk	1 c
Evaporated skim milk	½ c
Nonfat dry milk	⅓ c
Plain nonfat yogurt	1 c

Low-Fat Milk

2% milk	1 c
Vanilla low-fat yogurt (with added nonfat milk solids)	1 c

Whole Milk

The whole milk group has much more fat per serving than the skim and low-fat groups. Whole milk has more than 3¼ percent butterfat. Try to limit your choices from the whole milk group as much as possible.

Whole milk	1 c
Evaporated whole milk	½ c
Whole plain yogurt	1 c

FAT LIST

Each serving on the Fat List contains about 5 grams of fat and 45 calories.

The foods on this list contain mostly fat, although some items may also contain a small amount of protein. All fats are high in calories and should be carefully measured. You should modify fat intake by eating unsaturated fats instead of saturated fats. The sodium content of these foods varies widely. Check the label for sodium information.

Unsaturated Fats

Avocado	⅛ medium
Margarine	1 t
**Margarine, dietetic	1 T
Mayonnaise	1 t
**Mayonnaise, reduced-calorie	1 T
Nuts and seeds:	
Almonds, dry roasted	6 whole
Cashews, dry roasted	1 T
Pecans	2 whole
Peanuts	20 small or 10 large
Walnuts	2 whole
Other nuts	1T
Seeds, pine nuts, sunflower (without shells)	1 T
Pumpkin seeds	2 t
Oil (corn, cottonseed, safflower, soybean, sunflower, olive, peanut)	1 t
**Olives	10 small or 5 large
Salad dressing, mayonnaise-type	2 t
Salad dressing, mayonnaise-type, reduced-calorie	1 T
**Salad dressing (all varieties)	1 T
†Salad dressing, reduced-calorie	2 T

(Two tablespoons of low-calorie salad dressing is a free food.)

**If more than 1 or 2 servings are eaten, these foods have 400 mg or more of sodium.
†Indicates 400 mg or more of sodium

Saturated Fats

Butter	1 t
**Bacon	1 slice
Chitterlings	½ oz
Coconut, shredded	2 T
Coffee whitener, liquid	2 T
Coffee whitener, powder	4 t
Cream (heavy, whipping)	1 T
Cream (light)	2 T
Cream, sour	2 T
Cream cheese	1 T
**Salt pork	¼ oz

FREE FOODS

A *free food* is any food or drink that contains less than 20 calories per serving. You can eat as much as you want of those items that have no serving size specified. You may eat two or three servings per day of those items that have a specific serving size. Be sure to spread them out through the day.

Drinks

†Bouillon or broth without fat
Bouillon, low-sodium
Carbonated drinks, sugar-free
Carbonated water
Club soda
Cocoa powder, unsweetened (1 T)
Coffee/Tea
Drink mixes, sugar-free
Tonic water, sugar-free

Nonstick vegetable spray

Fruit

Cranberries, unsweetened (½ c)
Rhubarb, unsweetened (½ c)

**If more than 1 or 2 servings are eaten, these foods have 400 mg or more of sodium
†Indicates 400 mg or more of sodium

Vegetables *(raw, 1 c)*

Cabbage
Celery
*Chinese cabbage
Cucumber
Green onion
Hot peppers
Mushrooms
Radishes
*Zucchini

Salad greens

Endive
Escarole
Lettuce
Spinach

Sweet substitutes

Candy, hard, sugar-free
Gelatin, sugar-free
Gum, sugar-free
Jam/Jelly, dietetic (2 t)
Pancake syrup, sugar-free (1–2 T)
Sugar substitutes (saccharin, aspartame)
Whipped topping (2 T)

Condiments

Catsup (1 T)
Horseradish
Mustard
†Pickles, dill, unsweetened
Salad dressing, low-calorie (2 T)
Taco sauce (1 T)
Vinegar

Seasonings can be very helpful in making food taste better. Be aware of how much sodium you use. Read labels and choose seasonings that do not contain sodium or salt.

Allspice	Celery seeds	Chives
Basil (fresh)	Chili powder	Cinnamon

*Indicates 3 g or more of fiber
†Indicates 400 mg or more of sodium

Cloves	Hot pepper sauce	Pepper
Curry	Lemon	Pimiento
Dill	Lemon juice	Spices
Flavoring extracts (vanilla, almond, walnut, peppermint, butter, lemon, etc.)	Lemon pepper	†Soy sauce
	Lime	Soy sauce, low sodium ("lite")
	Lime juice	
	Mint	Wine, used in cooking (¼ c)
Garlic	Nutmeg	
Garlic powder	Onion powder	Worcestershire sauce
Herbs	Oregano	
	Paprika	

COMBINATION FOODS

Much of the food we eat is mixed together in various combinations. These combination foods do not fit into only one exchange list. It can be quite hard to tell what is in a certain casserole dish or baked food item. This list of average values for some typical combination foods will help you fit these foods into your meal plan. Ask your dietitian for information about other foods you'd like to eat.

Food	Amount	Exchanges
Casseroles, homemade	1 c	2 starch/bread, 2 medium-fat meat, 1 fat
†Cheese pizza, thin crust	¼ of 15 oz or ¼ of 10 in.	2 starch/bread, 1 medium-fat meat, 1 fat
*†Chili with beans (commercial)	1 c	2 starch/bread, 2 medium-fat meat, 2 fat
*†Chow mein (without noodles or rice)	2 c	1 starch/bread, 2 vegetable, 2 lean meat
†Macaroni and cheese	1 c	2 starch/bread, 1 medium-fat meat, 2 fat
Soup:		
*†Bean	1 c	1 starch/bread, 1 vegetable, 1 lean meat
†Chunky, all varieties	10¾-oz can	1 starch/bread, 1 vegetable, 1 medium-fat meat
†Cream (made with water)	1 c	1 starch/bread, 1 fat

*Indicates 3 g or more of fiber
†Indicates 400 mg or more of sodium

Food	Amount	Exchanges
†Vegetable or broth	1 c	1 starch/bread
†Spaghetti and meatballs (canned)	1 c	2 starch/bread, 1 medium-fat meat, 1 fat
Sugar-free pudding (made with skim milk)	½ c	1 starch/bread
If beans are used as a meat substitute:		
*Dried beans, peas, lentils	1 c (cooked)	2 starch/bread, 1 lean meat

FOODS FOR OCCASIONAL USE

Moderate amounts of some foods can be used in your meal plan, in spite of their sugar or fat content, as long as you can maintain blood-glucose control. The following list includes average exchange values for some of these foods. Because they are concentrated sources of carbohydrate, you will notice that the portion sizes are very small. Check with your dietitian for advice on how often and when you can eat them.

Food	Amount	Exchanges
Angel food cake	1/12 cake	2 starch/bread
Cake, no icing	1/12 cake, or 3-in. square	2 starch/bread, 2 fat
Cookies	2 small (1¾-in. across)	1 starch/bread, 1 fat
Frozen fruit yogurt	⅓ c	1 starch/bread
Gingersnaps	3	1 starch/bread
Granola	¼ c	1 starch/bread, 1 fat
Granola bars	1 small	1 starch/bread, 1 fat
Ice cream, any flavor	½ c	1 starch/bread, 2 fat
Ice milk, any flavor	½ c	1 starch/bread, 1 fat
Sherbert, any flavor	¼ c	1 starch/bread
†Snack chips, all varieties	1 oz	1 starch/bread, 2 fat
Vanilla wafers	6 small	1 starch/bread

*Indicates 3 g or more of fiber
†Indicates 400 mg or more of sodium

GLOSSARY OF
DIETARY TERMS

Beta cells   Found in the islets of Langerhans of the pancreas, these cells are where insulin is produced and released to maintain normal blood sugar levels.

Calorie   The term used to describe the energy value of foods (carbohydrate, protein, fat, and alcohol). It is the heat required to raise the temperature of 1 gram of water 1 degree. Also called a kilocalorie.

Carbohydrates   A major energy source, they are made by all plants from carbon, hydrogen, and oxygen, and provide 4 calories per gram. Carbohydrates are divided into monosaccharides, disaccharides, and polysaccharides.

Cholesterol   A type of fat that is a component of animal cells and is made within the body. Animal fats that are high in cholesterol tend to raise blood cholesterol levels. A healthy cholesterol level is below 200 mg/dl.

Cholesterol–Saturated Fat Index   The table developed by William and Sonja Connor in *The New American Diet* (Simon & Schuster, 1986), which considers saturated fat and cholesterol in foods. The lower the CSI number, the better the food choice.

Diabetes mellitus   A condition in which the body does not properly utilize carbohydrates for energy. A lack of insulin production or a defect in its action can cause diabetes mellitus.

Fat   The most calorically dense energy source, fat provides 9 calories per gram.

Fat substitute   Formulated with proteins or sucrose polyester, products utilizing this type of fat will allow consumers to enjoy the taste and texture of rich, creamy foods without the calories of fat.

Fiber   Dietary fiber is a group of complex carbohydrates that cannot

354

be digested by the human intestinal enzymes. It is found in fruits, vegetables, and whole grains, and is often called "roughage" or "bulk." The two types of fiber include water soluble and water insoluble. Soluble fiber helps to control blood sugar and cholesterol and is found in legumes, fruits, and oat products. Insoluble fiber adds bulk, improves regularity, and is found in whole grain wheat products and vegetables.

Food exchange lists Food guides for people planning a controlled diet. They were developed to provide optimal nutrition for the diabetic while controlling carbohydrate, protein, fat, and calorie intake. Foods within each group may be interchanged for meal planning.

Fructose A naturally occurring sugar, it is found in fruits, vegetables, and honey. Fructose is the sweetest natural sugar and is 70 percent sweeter than sucrose.

Glucose A simple sugar that is the body's primary source of fuel; also called dextrose.

Glycogen Carbohydrate that is stored as a complex of glucose molecules in the liver and muscles. It is utilized during fasting or insulin reactions when it is broken down into individual glucose molecules for metabolism.

High-density lipoprotein (HDL) cholesterol A combination of fat and protein, HDL (the "good" cholesterol) has been found to remove and carry cholesterol away from the cells of the large blood vessels, thereby reducing the risk of heart disease. Regular exercise increases this cholesterol.

Hyperglycemia Blood sugar levels above the normal range.

Hypertension High blood pressure that places increased strain on heart and blood vessels. Untreated, hypertension greatly increases risk for heart attack, stroke, and kidney disease.

Hypoglycemia Blood sugar below the normal range.

Insulin A hormone produced by beta cells in the pancreas. Its role is to help glucose get into your cells, where it can be used for energy.

Ketoacidosis Accumulation of ketones (end product of fat metabolism) in the body which increase the blood's acidity. Occurs when there is a lack of insulin and the body burns fat as the primary fuel. This condition, which occurs primarily in insulin-dependent people with diabetes, may lead to coma and death if untreated.

Ketone bodies By-products of fat metabolism, composed of acetone, acetoacetic acid, and betahydroxybutyric acid.

Low-density lipoprotein (LDL) cholesterol   A combination of fat and protein, LDL is called the "bad" cholesterol because it causes damage to the heart and blood vessels by depositing cholesterol in artery walls.

Monosaccharides   Rapidly absorbed simple sugars, which include glucose, fructose, and lactose, found in foods with high sugar content — jam, syrup, honey, etc.

Monounsaturated fat   An unsaturated fatty acid that appears to lower plasma cholesterol levels. Rich sources include olive oil, canola oil, and peanut oil.

Omega-3 fatty acid   Highly polyunsaturated fatty acid found in fish oil. Rich sources include shellfish, salmon, and mackerel.

Oral hypoglycemic agent   Medication that helps to lower blood sugar by stimulating the pancreas to produce more insulin.

Pancreas   A gland that secretes hormones such as insulin, glucagon, and somatostatin.

Polysaccharides   A long chain of slowly absorbed carbohydrates, found in legumes, vegetables, grains, and cereals.

Polyunsaturated fat   Widely known as essential fatty acids, which are necessary for a variety of bodily functions. Fats of vegetable origin, including corn and safflower oil, unhydrogenated soft shortenings, and soft margarines fall into this category. This type of fat tends to lower blood cholesterol levels.

Protein   Composed of amino acids, proteins are the "building blocks" of cells and are responsible for tissue growth and repair.

P:S ratio   Relationship between polyunsaturated and saturated fats in the diet. To obtain the ideal ratio of 1:0 requires a decrease in saturated fats.

Saturated fat   This type of fat is usually solid at room temperature. It is found primarily in foods of animal origin such as beef, lamb, and pork, and in the vegetable fats, palm and coconut oils, and cocoa butter. These fatty acids tend to increase blood cholesterol levels.

Sodium   Largely found in table salt, which is 40 percent sodium by weight, it occurs in many foods naturally and is an added ingredient to processed foods.

Sucrose   A disaccharide that is composed of glucose and fructose. Also called granulated sugar or table sugar.

GLOSSARY OF FOOD AND COOKING TERMS

Amaranth A grain rich in protein, calcium, iron, and phosphorus. Amaranth flour may be substituted for wheat flour with 1 part amaranth to 3 or 4 parts wheat flour.

Balsamic vinegar Aged for ten years in wooden barrels from Italy, this slightly sweet, full-bodied gourmet vinegar is reddish brown in color. It can be found in specialty shops and in some grocery stores.

Basmati rice Nutty-flavored long-grain white rice found in gourmet or specialty stores and Indian markets.

Blackened A cooking style popularized by Cajun cuisine. Preparation usually incorporates use of seasoned meat or fish cooked over very high temperatures in a hot iron skillet to achieve a black color.

Bulgur Whole wheat that has been cooked, dried, partly debranned, and cracked. Cooked, ⅓ c = 1 starch/bread exchange.

Cayenne A seasoning of chili peppers and salt, the word comes from Cayenne Island in French Guiana. Often used to spice up Mexican and Southern cooking.

Chicken broth, defatted Homemade or canned chicken broth that is chilled and has the fat layer skimmed off the top.

Chili peppers The chili family varies in flavor and hotness. Anaheim or California green chilies are among the mildest. The hottest chilies include the short Fresno, jalapeño, and serrano. Peppers are a rich source of vitamin C, and red peppers contain vitamin A as well.

Cilantro Mexican parsley, the fresh leaves of the coriander plant.

Equal The low-calorie sweetener containing NutraSweet, an ingredient composed of the two protein components phenylalanine and aspartic acid. One package of Equal (4 calories) = 2 teaspoons sugar (32 calories).

Knead   The method of developing gluten from wheat by manipulating dough on a floured surface.

Marinate   The process of thoroughly immersing foods in a liquid, usually to increase tenderness or enhance flavors.

Oat bran   The outer protective covering of the oat grain. One ounce dry contains 7 grams of dietary fiber and 110 calories.

Olive oil   Oil that has been pressed from olives and is a good source of monounsaturated fats. Extra virgin olive oil comes from the first pressing of the olive. The majority of olive oil is imported from the Mediterranean region.

Pita bread   Often called pocket bread, Sahara bread, or Arabian bread, it is a round, flat bread that is sliced open to form a pocket, then filled with meat or vegetables.

Reduced-calorie mayonnaise   Mayonnaise that is lower in fat and half the calories of regular mayonnaise; 1 tablespoon = 1 fat exchange.

Sauté   The method used traditionally to cook food in a small amount of fat. Newer low-calorie methods utilize liquid (water, wine, or broth) to replace the fat.

Tahini   A Middle Eastern specialty spread that is made from pulverized sesame seeds; 1 teaspoon = 1 fat exchange.

Tempeh   Fermented, boiled soybeans, bound together to form a firm cake that is seasoned and cooked.

Tofu   A soybean product made by curdling protein with calcium or magnesium salt. It has a soft or firm, smooth texture and a mild flavor. Tofu can be incorporated into a variety of recipes, from soups to dessert.

Tomatillo   A Mexican tomato that is small, green, and predominantly used in cooked sauces. It comes fresh or canned.

FOR FURTHER INFORMATION

American Association of Diabetes Educators
500 North Michigan Avenue, Suite 1400
Chicago, IL 60611
(312) 661-1700

American Diabetes Association
National Service Center
1660 Duke Street
Alexandria, VA 22314
(800) 232-3472

American Dietetic Association
Diabetes Care and Education Practice Group
216 West Jackson Boulevard, Suite 800
Chicago, IL 60606-6995
(312) 899-0040

Juvenile Diabetes Foundation International
432 Park Avenue South
New York, NY 10016
(212) 889-7575

National Diabetes Information Clearing House
Box NDIC
Bethesda, MD 20892
(301) 468-2162

INDEX